Mosby's
PHYSICAL
EXAMINATION
HANDBOOK

Mosby's
PHYSICAL EXAMINATION HANDBOOK

HENRY M. SEIDEL, M.D.
Professor of Pediatrics, School of Medicine
The Johns Hopkins University
Baltimore, Maryland

JANE W. BALL, R.N., C.P.N.P., Dr. P.H.
Director
Pediatric Emergency Education and Research Center
Children's National Medical Center
Washington, D.C.

JOYCE E. DAINS, R.N., Dr. P.H., J.D.
Former Associate Professor, School of Nursing
The University of Texas–Houston Health Science Center
Houston, Texas

G. WILLIAM BENEDICT, M.D., Ph.D.
Assistant Professor, School of Medicine
The Johns Hopkins University
Baltimore, Maryland

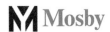 Mosby

St. Louis   Baltimore   Berlin   Boston   Carlsbad   Chicago   London   Madrid
Naples   New York   Philadelphia   Sydney   Tokyo   Toronto

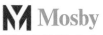
Mosby
Dedicated to Publishing Excellence

Publisher: Nancy Coon
Editor: Sally Schrefer
Developmental Editors: Penny Rudolph/Gail Brower
Developmental Writer: Tom Lochhaas
Project Manager: Patricia Tannian
Senior Production Editor: Ann E. Rogers
Senior Book Designer: Gail Morey Hudson
Manufacturing Supervisor: Kathy Grone
Cover Designer: Teresa Breckwoldt

Printed in the United States of America
Composition by The Clarinda Company
Printing/binding by Von Hoffmann Press, Inc.

Mosby–Year Book, Inc.
11830 Westline Industrial Drive
St. Louis, Missouri 63146

Library of Congress Cataloging in Publication Data

Mosby's physical examination handbook / Henry M. Seidel . . . [et al.].
    p.   cm.
    Includes bibliographical references and index.
    ISBN 0-8151-7820-4   (pbk.)
    1. Physical diagnosis—Handbooks, manuals, etc. I. Seidel, Henry
M. II. Title: Physical examination handbook.
    [DNLM: 1. Physical Examination—methods—handbooks. WB 39
1995]
RC76.M64   1995
616.07`5—dc20
DNLM/DLC
for Library of Congress   94-42785
                                                CIP

96 97 98 / 9 8 7 6 5 4 3 2

....

Contents

....

Introduction

Mosby's Physical Examination Handbook is a portable clinical reference on physical examination suitable for students of nursing, medicine, chiropractic, and other allied health disciplines, as well as practicing health care providers. It offers brief descriptions of examination techniques and guidelines on how the examination should proceed step by step. This text is intended to be an aid to review and recall the procedures for physical examination.

The text begins with an outline of what information should be obtained for the patient's medical history and gives a brief review of the body systems. Subsequent chapters for each of the body systems list equipment needed to perform the examination and present the techniques to be used. Expected and unexpected findings follow the description of each technique. More than 180 illustrations interspersed throughout the text reinforce recall of techniques and possible findings. Each chapter offers aids to differential diagnosis and also provides sample documentation.

The two final chapters of the text give an overview of the entire examination—head to toe—and give guidelines for reporting and recording findings.

1

....

The History

TAKING THE HISTORY

The following outline of what to include when taking a patient history should be viewed not as a rigid structure but a general guideline. Since you are beginning your relationship with the patient at this point, pay attention to this relationship as well as to the information you seek in the history. Be friendly and show respect for the patient. Choose a comfortable setting and help the patient get settled. Maintain eye contact and use a conversational tone. Begin by introducing yourself and explaining your role. Help the patient understand why you are taking the history and how it will be used. Once the history proceeds, explore positive responses with additional questions: where, when, what, how, and why. Be sensitive to the patient's emotions at all times.

CHIEF COMPLAINT

The problem or symptom: reason for visit
Duration of problem
Patient information: age, sex, marital status; previous hospital admissions; occupation
Other complaints: secondary issues, fears, concerns; what made the patient seek care

PRESENT PROBLEM

Chronologic ordering: sequence of events patient has experienced
State of health just before the onset of the present problem
Complete description of the first symptom: time and date of onset, location, movement
Possible exposure to infection or toxic agents

If symptoms intermittent, describe typical attack: onset, duration, symptoms, variations, inciting factors, exacerbating factors, relieving factors

Impact of illness: on lifestyle, on ability to function, limitations
imposed by illness

"Stability" of the problem: intensity variations, improvement,
worsening, staying the same

Immediate reason for seeking attention, particularly for long-
standing problem

Review of appropriate system when there is a conspicuous disturbance of a particular organ or system

Medications: current and recent, dosage of prescriptions, home
remedies, nonprescription medications

Review of chronology of events for each problem: patient's con-
firmations and corrections

PAST MEDICAL HISTORY

General health and strength

Childhood illnesses: measles, mumps, whooping cough, chicken
pox, smallpox, scarlet fever, acute rheumatic fever, diphtheria,
poliomyelitis

Major adult illnesses: tuberculosis, hepatitis, diabetes, hypertension, myocardial infarction, tropical or parasitic diseases,
other infections, any nonsurgical hospital admissions

Immunizations: poliomyelitis, diphtheria, pertussis, and tetanus
toxoid, influenza, cholera, typhus, typhoid, bacille Calmette-
Guérin (BCG), HBV, last PPD or other skin tests; unusual reactions to immunizations; tetanus or other antitoxin made with
horse serum

Surgery: dates, hospital, diagnosis, complications

Serious injuries: resulting disability (document fully for injuries
with possible legal implications)

Limitation of ability to function as desired as a result of past
events

Medications: past, current and recent medications; dosage of
prescription; home remedies and nonprescription medications

Allergies: especially to medications, but also to environmental
allergens and foods

Transfusions: reactions, date, and number of units transfused

Emotional status: mood disorders, psychiatric treatment

Children: birth, developmental milestones, childhood diseases, immunizations

FAMILY HISTORY

Relatives with similar illness

Immediate family: ethnicity, health, cause of and age at death

History of disease: heart disease, high blood pressure, hypercholesterolemia, cancer, tuberculosis, stroke, epilepsy, diabetes, gout, kidney disease, thyroid disease, asthma and other allergic states; forms of arthritis; blood diseases; sexually transmitted diseases; other familial diseases

Spouse and children: age, health

Hereditary disease: history of grandparents, aunts, uncles, siblings, cousins; consanguinity

PERSONAL AND SOCIAL HISTORY

Personal status: birthplace, where raised; home environment: parental divorce or separation, socioeconomic class, cultural background; education; position in family; marital status; general life satisfaction; hobbies and interests; sources of stress and strain

Habits: nutrition and diet, regularity and patterns of eating and sleeping; exercise: quantity and type; quantity of coffee, tea, tobacco; alcohol; illicit drugs: frequency, type amount; breast or testicular self-examination

Sexual history: concerns with sexual feelings and performance; frequency of intercourse, ability to achieve orgasm, number and variety of partners

Home conditions: housing, economic condition, type of health insurance if any; pets and their health

Occupation: description of usual work and present work if different; list of job changes; work conditions and hours; physical and mental strain; duration of employment; present and past exposure to heat and cold, industrial toxins, especially lead, arsenic, chromium, asbestos, beryllium, poisonous gases, benzene, and polyvinyl chloride or other carcinogens and teratogens; any protective devices required, for example, goggles or masks

Environment: travel and other exposure to contagious diseases, residence in tropics, water and milk supply, other sources of infection if applicable

Military record: dates and geographic area of assignments

Religious preference: determine any religious proscriptions concerning medical care

Cost of care: resources available to patient, financial worries, candid discussion of issues

REVIEW OF SYSTEMS

General constitutional symptoms: fever, chills, malaise, fatigability, night sweats; weight (average, preferred, present, change)

Diet: appetite, likes and dislikes, restrictions (because of religion, allergy, or disease), vitamins and other supplements, use of caffeine-containing beverages (coffee, tea, cola); an hour-by-hour detailing of food and liquid intake—sometimes a written diary covering several days of intake may be necessary

Skin, hair, and nails: rash or eruption, itching, pigmentation or texture change; excessive sweating, abnormal nail or hair growth; in children, eczema or seborrhea

Musculoskeletal: joint stiffness, pain, restriction of motion, swelling, redness, heat, bony deformity

Head and neck:

General: frequent or unusual headaches, their location, dizziness, syncope, severe head injuries; periods of loss of consciousness (momentary or prolonged)

Eyes: visual acuity, blurring, diplopia, photophobia, pain, recent change in appearance or vision; glaucoma, use of eye drops or other eye medications; history of trauma or familial eye disease

Ears: hearing loss, pain, discharge, tinnitus, vertigo; in children, otitis media

Nose: sense of smell, frequency of colds, obstruction, epistaxis, postnasal discharge, sinus pain; in children, mouth breathing

Throat and mouth: hoarseness or change in voice; frequent sore throats, bleeding or swelling of gums; recent tooth abscesses or extractions; soreness of tongue or buccal mucosa, ulcers; disturbance of taste

Endocrine: thyroid enlargement or tenderness, heat or cold intolerance, unexplained weight change, diabetes, polydipsia, polyuria, changes in facial or body hair, increased hat and glove size, skin striae

Males: puberty onset, erections, emissions, testicular pain, libido, infertility

Females:

Menses: onset, regularity, duration and amount of flow, dysmenorrhea, last period, intermenstrual discharge or bleeding, itching, date of last Pap smear, age at menopause, libido, frequency of intercourse, sexual difficulties, infertility

Pregnancies: number, miscarriages, abortions, duration of pregnancy, each type of delivery, any complications during any pregnancy or postpartum period or with neonate; use of oral or other contraceptives

Breasts: pain, tenderness, discharge, lumps, galactorrhea, mammograms (screening or diagnostic), frequency of breast self-examination

Chest and lungs: pain related to respiration, dyspnea, cyanosis, wheezing, cough, sputum (character and quantity), hemoptysis, night sweats, exposure to TB; date and result of last chest x-ray examination

Heart and blood vessels: chest pain or distress, precipitating causes, timing and duration, character; relieving factors; palpitations, dyspnea, orthopnea (number of pillows needed), edema, claudication, hypertension, previous myocardial infarction, estimate of exercise tolerance, past ECG or other cardiac tests

Hematologic: anemia, tendency to bruise or bleed easily, thromboses, thrombophlebitis, any known abnormality of blood cells, transfusions

Lymph nodes: enlargement, tenderness, suppuration

Gastrointestinal: appetite, digestion, intolerance for any class of foods, dysphagia, heartburn, nausea, vomiting, hematemesis, regularity of bowels, constipation, diarrhea, change in stool color or contents (clay-colored, tarry, fresh blood, mucus, undigested food), flatulence, hemorrhoids, hepatitis, jaundice, dark urine; history of ulcer, gallstones, polyps, tumor; previous x-ray examinations (where, when, findings)

Genitourinary: dysuria, flank or suprapubic pain, urgency, frequency, nocturia, hematuria, polyuria, hesitancy, dribbling, loss in force of stream, passage of stone; edema of face, stress incontinence, hernias, sexually transmitted disease (inquire type and symptoms, and results of serologic test for syphilis, if known)

Neurologic: syncope, seizures, weakness or paralysis, abnormalities of sensation or coordination, tremors, loss of memory

Psychiatric: depression, mood changes, difficulty concentrating, nervousness, tension, suicidal thoughts, irritability, sleep disturbances

....

2

Skin, Hair, and Nails

EQUIPMENT

♦ Centimeter ruler (flexible, clear)
♦ Wood's lamp
♦ Flashlight with transilluminator
♦ Magnifying glass (optional)

EXAMINATION

TECHNIQUE	FINDINGS

Skin

Perform visual sweep of entire body

In particular, check areas not usually exposed and intertriginous surfaces.

Expected: Skin color differences among body areas and between sun-exposed and non–sun-exposed areas.
Unexpected: Lesions.

Inspect skin of each body area

and mucous membranes

♦ Color/uniformity
Inspect sclerae, conjunctivae, buccal mucosa, tongue, lips, nail beds, and palms of dark-skinned patients for color hues.

Expected: General uniformity: dark brown to light tan, with pink or yellow overtones. Sun-darkened areas. Darker skin around knees and elbows. Calloused areas yellow. Knuckles darker and palms/soles lighter in dark-skinned patients. Vascular-flush areas pink or red, especially with anxiety or excitement. Pigmented nevi. Nonpigmented striae. Freckles. Birthmarks.

VASCULAR SKIN LESIONS

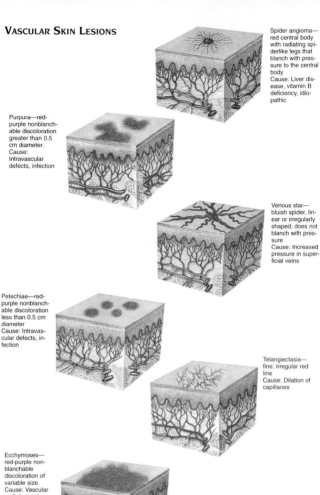

Spider angioma—red central body with radiating spiderlike legs that blanch with pressure to the central body
Cause: Liver disease, vitamin B deficiency, idiopathic

Purpura—red-purple nonblanchable discoloration greater than 0.5 cm diameter.
Cause: Intravascular defects, infection

Venous star—bluish spider, linear or irregularly shaped; does not blanch with pressure
Cause: Increased pressure in superficial veins

Petechiae—red-purple nonblanchable discoloration less than 0.5 cm diameter
Cause: Intravascular defects, infection

Telangiectasia—fine, irregular red line
Cause: Dilation of capillaries

Ecchymoses—red-purple nonblanchable discoloration of variable size
Cause: Vascular wall destruction, trauma, vasculitis

Capillary hemangioma (nevus flammeus)—red irregular macular patches
Cause: Dilation of dermal capillaries

TECHNIQUE	FINDINGS
	Unexpected: Dysplastic, precancerous, or cancerous nevi. Chloasma. Unpigmented skin. Generalized or localized color changes. Vascular skin lesions.
◆ Thickness	Expected: Thickness variations, with eyelids thinnest, areas of rubbing thickest. Calluses on hands and feet.
◆ Symmetry	Expected: Bilateral symmetry.
◆ Hygiene In children inspect hand and foot creases.	Expected: Clean. *Unexpected: Simian line.*

Palpate skin

◆ Moisture	Expected: Minimal perspiration or oiliness. Increased perspiration (associated with activity, environment, obesity, anxiety, and excitement) noticeable on palms, scalp, forehead, and axillae. *Unexpected: Damp intertriginous areas.*
◆ Temperature Palpate with dorsal surface of hand or fingers.	Expected: Cool to warm. Bilateral symmetry.
◆ Texture	Expected: Smooth, soft, and even. Roughness resulting from heavy clothing, cold weather, or soap. *Unexpected: Extensive or widespread roughness.*
◆ Turgor and mobility Gently pinch skin on forearm or in sternal area and release.	Expected: Resilience. *Unexpected: Failure of skin to return to place quickly.*

TECHNIQUE	FINDINGS

Inspect and palpate lesions

♦ Size
  Measure all dimensions.

Unexpected: See figures on pp. 11-12.

♦ Shape/configuration
♦ Color
  Use Wood's lamp to distinguish fluorescing lesions
♦ Blanching
♦ Texture
  Transilluminate to determine presence of fluid.
♦ Elevation/depression
♦ Pedunculation
♦ Exudates
  Note color, odor, amount, and consistency of lesion.
♦ Pattern
  Check lesion for annular, grouped, linear, arciform, or diffuse arrangement.
♦ Location/distribution
  Check lesion for generalized/localized, body region, patterns (dermatomal, flexor/extensor, random, or clothing- or jewelry-related), or discrete/confluent.

PRIMARY SKIN LESIONS

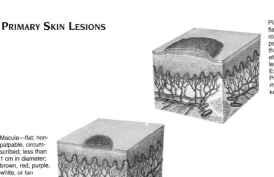

Plaque—elevated, flat topped, firm, rough, superficial papule greater than 1 cm in diameter; may be coalesced papules
Examples: Psoriasis; seborrheic and actinic keratoses

Macule—flat; nonpalpable, circumscribed; less than 1 cm in diameter; brown, red, purple, white, or tan
Examples: Freckles; flat moles; rubella; rubeola

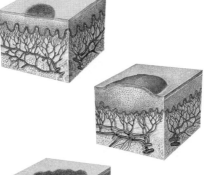

Wheal—elevated, irregular-shaped area of cutaneous edema; solid, transient, changing, variable diameter; pale pink with lighter center
Examples: Urticaria; insect bites

Patch—flat, nonpalpable, irregular in shape; macule that is greater than 1 cm in diameter
Examples: Vitiligo; port-wine marks

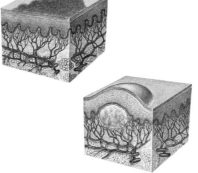

Nodule—elevated, firm, circumscribed, palpable; deeper in dermis than papule; 1 to 2 cm in diameter
Examples: Erythema nodosum; lipomas

Papule—elevated, palpable, firm, circumscribed; less than 1 cm in diameter; brown, red, pink, tan, or bluish red in color
Examples: Warts; drug-related eruptions; pigmented nevi

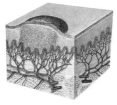

PRIMARY SKIN LESIONS—cont'd

Tumor—elevated; solid; may or may not be clearly demarcated; greater than 2 cm in diameter; may or may not vary from skin color
Example: Neoplasms

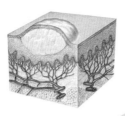

Pustule—elevated; superficial; similar to vesicle but filled with purulent fluid
Examples: Impetigo; acne; variola

Vesicle—elevated; circumscribed; superficial; filled with serous fluid; less than 1 cm in diameter
Examples: Blister; varicella

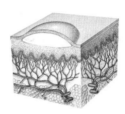

Cyst—elevated; circumscribed; palpable; encapsulated; filled with liquid or semisolid material
Example: Sebaceous cyst

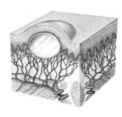

Bulla—vesicle greater than 1 cm in diameter
Examples: Blister; pemphigus vulgaris

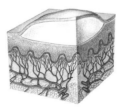

TECHNIQUE	FINDINGS

Hair
Inspect hair over entire body

♦ Color

Expected: Light blond to black and gray, with alterations caused by rinses, dyes, and permanents.

♦ Distribution/quantity

Expected: Hair present on scalp, lower face, neck, nares, ears, chest, axillae, back and shoulders, arms, legs, pubic areas, and around nipples. Scalp hair loss in adult men, adrenal androgenic female-pattern alopecia in adult women.
Unexpected: Localized or generalized hair loss. Inflammation or scarring. Broken/absent hair shafts. Hirsutism in women.

Palpate for texture

Expected: Coarse or fine, curly or straight, shiny, smooth, and resilient. Fine vellus covering body; coarse terminal hair on scalp, pubic, and axillary areas and in male beard.
Unexpected: Dryness and brittleness.

Nails
Inspect nails

♦ Color

Expected: Variations of pink with varying opacity. Pigment deposits in persons with dark skin. White spots.
Unexpected: Yellow or green-black discoloration. Diffuse darkening. Pigment deposits in persons with light skin. Longitudinal red, brown, or white streaks, or white bands. White, yellow, or green tinge.

TECHNIQUE	**FINDINGS**
♦ Length/configuration/ symmetry	**Expected:** Varying shape, smooth and flat/slightly convex, with edges smooth and rounded. *Unexpected: Jagged, broken, or bitten edges or cuticles. Peeling. Absence of nail.*
♦ Cleanliness	**Expected:** Clean and neat. *Unexpected: Unkempt.*
♦ Ridging and beading	**Expected:** Longitudinal ridging and beading. *Unexpected: Longitudinal ridging and grooving with lichen planus. Transverse grooving, rippling, and depressions. Pitting.*

Palpate nail plate

♦ Texture/firmness/ thickness/uniformity	**Expected:** Hard and smooth with uniform thickness. *Unexpected: Thickening or thinning.*
♦ Adherence to nail bed Gently squeeze between thumb and finger.	**Expected:** Firmness. *Unexpected: Separation. Boggy nail base.*

Measure nail base angle

Inspect fingers when patient places dorsal surfaces of fingertips together.	**Expected:** 160-degree angle. *Unexpected: Clubbing.*

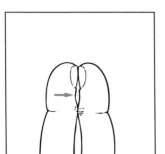

Expected finding

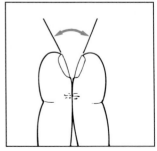

Clubbing

TECHNIQUE	FINDINGS
Inspect and palpate proximal and lateral nail fold	*Unexpected*: *Redness, swelling, pus, warts, cysts, tumors, and pain.*

AIDS TO DIFFERENTIAL DIAGNOSIS

ABNORMALITY	DESCRIPTION
Corn (clavus)	Flat or slightly elevated, circumscribed, painful lesions. Smooth, hard surface. Soft corns: whitish thickenings. Hard corns: sharply delineated, conical.
Callus	Superficial area of hyperkeratosis. Less demarcated than corns. Usually nontender.
Tinea (dermatophytosis)	Papular, pustular, vesicular, erythematous, or scaling lesions. Possible secondary bacterial infection.
Basal cell carcinoma	Cutaneous neoplasm in nodular, pigmented, cystic, sclerosing, superficial, and other forms.
Kaposi sarcoma	Soft, vascular, bluish purple, painless lesions. Macular or papular. May appear as plaques, keloids, or ecchymotic areas.
Eczematous dermatitis	Acute: erythematous, pruritic, weeping vesicles, often excoriated and crusted from scratching. Subacute: erythema and scaling, possible itching. Chronic: thick, lichenified, pruritic plaques.
Paronychia	Redness, swelling, tenderness at lateral and proximal nail

ABNORMALITY	DESCRIPTION
	folds. Possible purulent drainage under cuticle. Acute or chronic (with nail rippling).
Ingrown nail	Pain and swelling resulting from nail piercing fold and growing into dermis.
Abnormalities in children	
Café au lait patches	Coffee colored multiple patches, diameter >1 cm.
Seborrheic dermatitis	Thick, yellow, adherent crusted scalp, ear, or neck lesions.
Impetigo	Honey-colored crusted or ruptured vesicles.

SAMPLE DOCUMENTATION

Skin. Dark brown, soft, moist, warm; turgor: resilient, returns to place immediately; no edema, odor, or excess perspiration; freckling over cheeks and nose; 2 cm scar over right scapula, no keloid; no lesions.

Hair. Coarse, curly, black mixed with gray; male distribution patterns; thinning on crown; no infestation.

Nails. Nail plate smooth, hard, uniform, with longitudinal pigmented bands; nail base angle 160 degrees; nail bed firmly adhered; nail folds without redness, tenderness, lesions.

CHAPTER

3

·····

Lymphatic System

EQUIPMENT

♦ Centimeter ruler
♦ Skin-marking pencil

EXAMINATION

The lymphatic system is examined by inspection and palpation, region by region, during the examination of other body systems, as well as with palpation of the spleen.

THE LYMPH NODES MOST ACCESSIBLE TO INSPECTION AND PALPATION

Obviously, the more superficial the node, the more accessible.

The "Necklace" of Nodes

Parotid and retropharyngeal (tonsillar)
Submandibular
Submental
Sublingual (facial)
Superficial anterior cervical
Superficial posterior cervical
Preauricular and postauricular
Sternomastoid
Occipital
Supraclavicular

The Arms

Axiliary
Epitrochlear (cubital)

The Legs

Superficial superior inguinal
Superficial inferior inguinal
Occasionally, popliteal

TECHNIQUE	FINDINGS

Head and Neck

Inspect visible nodes

Ask if patient is aware of any lumps.

Unexpected: Edema, erythema, red streaks, or lesions.

Palpate for superficial nodes; note size, consistency, mobility, tenderness, warmth

Bend patient's head slightly forward or to the side. Palpate gently with pads of second, third, and fourth fingers.

Preauricular
Postauricular
Occipital
Tonsillar
Facial
Submental
Submandibular
Superficial anterior deep cervical
Supraclavicular
Epitrochlear
Superficial posterior cervical
Axillary
Superficial superior inguinal
Superficial inferior inguinal

G. J. Wassilchenko

TECHNIQUE	FINDINGS
Head/Neck	**Expected:** Nodes accessible to palpation but not large or firm enough to be felt. In children, small, firm, discrete, nontender, nonmovable nodes in occipital, postauricular chains.
♦ Occipital nodes at base of skull	
♦ Postauricular nodes over mastoid process	
♦ Preauricular nodes in front of ears	
♦ Parotid and retropharyngeal nodes at angle of mandible	**Unexpected:** *Enlarged, tender, red or discolored, fixed, matted, inflamed, or warm nodes, and increased vascularity.*
♦ Submaxillary nodes between angle and tip of mandible	
♦ Submental nodes behind tip of mandible	
Neck	**Expected:** Nodes accessible to palpation but not large or firm enough to be felt.
♦ Superficial cervical nodes at sternocleidomastoid	

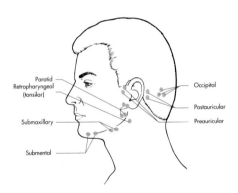

Parotid
Retropharyngeal
(tonsilar)

Submaxillary

Submental

Occipital

Postauricular

Preauricular

♦ Posterior cervical nodes along anterior border of trapezius

♦ Deep cervical nodes along anterior border of trapezius

Unexpected: *Enlarged, tender, red or discolored, fixed, matted, inflamed, or warm nodes, and increased vasculation.*

TECHNIQUE	**FINDINGS**

♦ Supraclavicular areas
If enlarged nodes are
found, inspect regions
drained by the nodes
for infection or malig-
nancy and examine
other regions for en-
largement.

Unexpected: Detection of Virchow nodes.

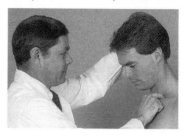

Axillae
Inspect visible nodes

Ask if patient is aware
of any lumps.

Unexpected: Edema, erythema, red
streaks, or lesions.

**Palpate superficial
nodes for size,
consistency, mobility,
tenderness, warmth**

Using firm, deliberate,
gentle touch, rotate
fingertips and palm.
Attempt to glide fin-
gers beneath nodes.

Axillary nodes
Support patient's fore-
arm with your con-
tralateral arm and
bring palm of examin-
ing hand flat into ax-
illa.

Expected: Nodes accessible to
palpation, but not large or firm
enough to be felt.
Unexpected: Enlarged, tender; red or
discolored; fixed, matted; inflamed, warm;
increased vascularity.

If enlarged nodes are
found, inspect regions
drained by the nodes
for infection or malig-
nancy and examine
other regions for en-
largement.

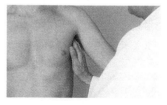

TECHNIQUE	FINDINGS

Other Lymph Nodes

Inspect visible nodes

Ask if patient is aware of any lumps.

Unexpected: Edema, erythema, red streaks, or lesions.

Palpate superficial nodes for size, consistency, mobility, tenderness, warmth

Systematically palpate other areas, moving hand in circular fashion, probing without pressing hard.

♦ Epitrochlear nodes Support elbow in one hand while exploring with the other.

Expected: Nodes accessible to palpation, but not large or firm enough to be felt.
Unexpected: Enlarged, tender; red or discolored; fixed, matted; inflamed, warm; increased vascularity.

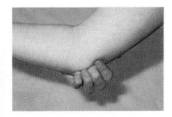

♦ Inguinal and popliteal area
Have patient lie supine with knee slightly flexed.

Expected: In children, small, firm, discrete nodes; nontender, non-movable in inguinal chain.

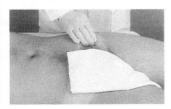

TECHNIQUE	FINDINGS
If enlarged nodes are found, inspect regions drained by the nodes for infection or malignancy and examine other regions for enlargement.	

AIDS TO DIFFERENTIAL DIAGNOSIS

ABNORMALITY	DESCRIPTION
Acute lymphangitis	Pain, malaise, illness, and possibly fever. Red streak (tracing of fine lines) may follow course of lymphatic collecting duct. Inflamed area sometimes slightly in durated and palpable to gentle touch. Related infection possible distally, particularly interdigitally.

SOME CONDITIONS SIMULATING LYMPH NODE ENLARGEMENT

Lymphangioma
Hemangioma (tends to feel spongy; appears reddish blue, depending on size and extent of angiomatous involvement)
Branchial cleft cyst (sometimes accompanied by a tiny orifice in the neck on a line extending to the ear)
Thyroglossal duct cyst
Laryngocele
Esophageal diverticulum
Thyroid goiter
Graves disease
Hashimoto thyroiditis
Parotid swelling (e.g., from mumps or tumor)

ABNORMALITY	DESCRIPTION
Non-Hodgkin lymphoma	Well-defined, solid neoplasm, often in lymph nodes or spleen.
Hodgkin disease	Painless, inexorably progressive enlargement of cervical lymph nodes. Generally asymmetric. Nodes sometimes matted and generally very firm, almost rubbery. Nodes sometimes produce pressure on surrounding structures, prompting need for medical care.
Epstein-Barr virus; mononucleosis	Pharyngitis, fever, fatigue, and malaise. Frequently splenomegaly. Occasionally hepatomegaly and/or rash. Palpable nodes generalized, but more commonly in anterior and posterior cervical chains. Nodes vary in firmness, are generally discrete, and are occasionally tender.
Streptococcal pharyngitis	Sore throat. Often runny nose. Sometimes headache, fatigue, and abdominal pain. Firm, discrete, often tender anterior cervical nodes generally felt.
Herpes simplex	Often discrete labial and gingival ulcers, high fever, and enlargement of anterior cervical and submandibular nodes. Nodes tend to be firm, quite discrete, movable, and tender.
Acquired immuno-deficiency syndrome (AIDS)	Recurrent, often severe, opportunistic infections. Initially: lymphadenopathy, fatigue, fever, and weight loss.

ABNORMALITY	DESCRIPTION
HIV seropositivity	Warning signs include severe fatigue, malaise, weakness, persistent unexplained weight loss, persistent lymphadenopathy, fevers, arthralgias, and persistent diarrhea.

SAMPLE DOCUMENTATION

No visible enlargement of lymph nodes in any area. On palpation, enlarged node (2 cm in diameter) in left posterior cervical triangle, firm, nontender, movable, no overlying warmth, erythema, or edema. In addition, a few shotty nodes palpated in posterior cervical triangles bilaterally and in femoral chains bilaterally.

CHAPTER

4

························

Head and Neck

EQUIPMENT

♦ Tape measure
♦ Stethoscope
♦ Cup of water
♦ Transilluminator

EXAMINATION

Ask patient to sit.

TECHNIQUE	FINDINGS
Head and Face	
Observe head position	*Expected:* Upright, midline, and still.
	Unexpected: Horizontal jerking or bobbing, nodding, tilted.
Inspect facial features	
♦ Shape Observe eyelids; eyebrows; palpebral fissures; nasolabial folds; and mouth at rest, during movement, and with expression.	*Expected:* Variations according to race, sex, and body build. *Unexpected: Change in shape. Unusual features: edema, puffiness, coarsened features, prominent eyes, hirsutism, lack of expression, excessive perspiration, pallor, or pigmentation variations. Tics.*
♦ Symmetry Note if asymmetry affects all features of one side or a portion of face.	*Expected:* Slight asymmetry. *Unexpected: Facial nerve paralysis, facial nerve weakness, or problem with peripheral trigeminal nerve.*
♦ Characteristic facies	

TECHNIQUE	FINDINGS

Inspect skull and scalp

♦ Size/shape/symmetry
♦ Scalp condition
  Systematically part
  hair from frontal to occipital region.
♦ Hair pattern
  Pay special attention
  to areas behind ears,
  at hairline, and at
  crown.

Expected: Symmetric.

Unexpected: *Lesions, scabs, tenderness, parasites, nits, scaliness. In infants: scaling and crusting.*

Expected: Bitemporal recession or balding over crown.

Palpate head and scalp

♦ Symmetry
  Palpate in gentle, ro-
  tary motion from front
  to back.

Expected: Symmetric and smooth with bones indistinguishable. Ridge of sagittal occasionally palpable. An infant's head circumference is 2 cm > chest circumference up to the age of 2 years.
Unexpected: *Indentations or depressions.*

  In infants, transilluminate the skull
♦ Skull condition

♦ Scalp

Expected: 2 cm ring of light.

Expected: In infants, posterior fontanels closed at birth; anterior fontanels closed at 18-24 months.
Unexpected: *Tenderness or depressions, sunken areas, swelling, bulging or depressed fontanels.*
Expected: Free movement.
Unexpected:

Percuss the skull in infants

Expected: Macewen sign, cracked-pot sound, is physiologic when fontanels are open, *but may indicate increased intracranial pressure after fontanel closure.*

TECHNIQUE	FINDINGS

Palpate hair

♦ Texture/color distribution

Expected: Smooth, symmetrically distributed.
Unexpected: Splitting, or cracked ends. Coarse, dry, or brittle. Fine and silky.

Palpate temporal arteries

Note course of arteries

Unexpected: Thickening, hardness, or tenderness.

Auscultate temporal arteries

Auscultate over skull and eyes

Expected: Bruits are common in children up to 5 years old.
Unexpected: Bruit.

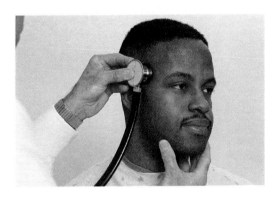

Inspect salivary glands

♦ Symmetry/size
Palpate if asymmetry noted. Have patient open mouth and press on the salivary duct to attempt to express material.

Unexpected: Asymmetry or enlargement. Tenderness. Discrete nodule.

TECHNIQUE	FINDINGS

Neck
Inspect neck

♦ Symmetry
Inspect in usual position, in slight hyperextension, and during swallowing. Look for landmarks of anterior and posterior triangles.

Expected: Bilateral symmetry of sternocleidomastoid and trapezius muscles.
Unexpected: *Asymmetry, torticollis.*

♦ Trachea
Inspect in usual position, in slight hyperextension, and while patient swallows.

Expected: Midline placement.

♦ Condition of neck

Unexpected: *Masses, webbing, excessive posterior skin folds, unusually short neck, distention of jugular vein, prominence of carotid arteries, or edema.*

Evaluate range of motion

Have patient flex, extend, rotate, and laterally turn head and neck.

Expected: Smooth.
Unexpected: *Pain or dizziness.*

Palpate neck

♦ Trachea
Place a thumb on each side of trachea in lower portion of neck, and compare space between trachea and sternocleidomastoid on each side.

Expected: Midline position.
Unexpected: *Deviation to right or left.*

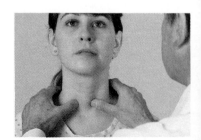

TECHNIQUE	FINDINGS
◆ Hyoid bone/thyroid and cricoid cartilages Have patient swallow.	**Expected:** Smooth. Moves during swallowing. *Unexpected: Tender.*
◆ Cartilaginous rings of trachea Have patient swallow.	**Expected:** Distinct. *Unexpected: Tender.*
◆ Tracheal tug With neck extended, palpate for movement with index finger and thumb on each side of trachea below thyroid isthmus.	*Unexpected: Downward tug synchronous with pulse.*

Palpate lymph nodes

◆ Size/consistency, mobility/condition	*Unexpected: Enlarged, matted, tender, fixed, warm.*

Palpate thyroid gland

◆ Symmetry Observe while patient hyperextends neck. Then observe while patient sips water while neck is hyperextended.	**Expected:** In children, thyroid gland may be palpable. *Unexpected: Asymmetry. Enlarged and visible thyroid gland.*

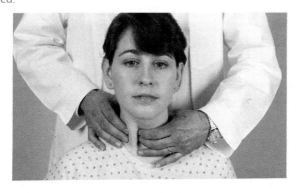

TECHNIQUE	FINDINGS
♦ Size/shape/configuration/consistency	
Stand either facing or behind patient. Have patient hold head slightly forward and tipped toward side being examined. Lightly palpate isthmus, main body, and lateral lobes. Give water to patient to facilitate swallowing.	**Expected:** Lobes (if felt) small and smooth. Gland rises freely with swallowing. Right lobe as much as 25% larger than left. Tissue firm and pliable. *Unexpected: Enlarged, tenderness, nodules (smooth or irregular, soft or hard), coarse tissue, and gritty sensation.*
If gland is enlarged, auscultate for vascular sounds with stethoscope bell.	**Unexpected:** Bruit.

AIDS TO DIFFERENTIAL DIAGNOSIS

ABNORMALITY	DESCRIPTION
Myxedema	Dull, puffy, yellow skin. Coarse, sparse hair. Temporal loss of eyebrows. Periorbital edema. Prominent tongue. Hypothyroidism (see p. 34).
Graves disease	Diffuse thyroid enlargement, hyperthyroidism. Various pathologic conditions: opthalmologic (prominent eyes, lid retraction, staring or startled expression), dermatologic (fine and moist skin, fine hair), and musculoskeletal (muscle weakness).
Down syndrome	Depressed nasal bridge, epicanthal folds, mongoloid slant of eyes, low-set ears, large tongue.

HEADACHES

Headaches are one of the most common complaints and probably one of the most self-medicated. They are not always benign. A history of insistent headache, severe and recurrent, must always be given attention. Sometimes the underlying cause is life threatening, such as a brain tumor. Sometimes it is life intimidating, such as migraines. At other times it is easily confronted, such as when it is the result of drinking wine. The patient's history is fully as important as the physical examination in getting at the root of a headache. Various kinds of headaches can be compared as follows.

Characteristic	Classic migraine	Common migraine	Cluster	Hypertensive	Muscular, tension	Temporal arteritis
Age at onset	Childhood	Childhood	Adulthood	Adulthood	Adulthood	Older adulthood
Location	Unilateral	Generalized	Unilateral	Bilateral or occipital	Unilateral or bilateral	Unilateral or bilateral
Duration	Hour to days	Hours to days	½ to 2 hours	Hours	Hours to days	Hours to days
Time of onset	Morning or night	Morning or night	Night	Morning	Anytime, commonly in afternoon or evening	Anytime

HEADACHES—cont'd

Characteristic	Classic migraine	Common migraine	Cluster	Hypertensive	Muscular, tension	Temporal arteritis
Quality of pain	Pulsating or throbbing	Pulsating or throbbing	Intense burning, boring, searing, knifelike	Throbbing	Bandlike, constricting	Throbbing
Prodromal event	Well-defined neurologic event, scotoma, aphasia, hemianopsia, aura	Vague neurologic changes, personality change, fluid retention, appetite loss	Personality changes, sleep disturbances	None	None	None
Precipitating event	Menstrual period, missing meals, birth control pills, let down after stress	Menstrual period, missing meals, birth control pills, let down after stress	Alcohol consumption	None	Stress, anger, bruxism	None

HEADACHES—cont'd

Characteristic	Classic migraine	Common migraine	Cluster	Hypertensive	Muscular, tension	Temporal arteritis
Frequency	Twice a week	Twice a week	Several times nightly for several nights, then none	Daily	Daily	Daily
Gender predilection	Females	Females	Males	Equal	Equal	Equal
Other Symptoms	Nausea, vomiting	Nausea, vomiting	Increased lacrimation, nasal discharge	Generally remits as day progresses	None	None

HYPERTHYROIDISM VERSUS HYPOTHYROIDISM

System or structure Affected	Hyperthyroidism	Hypothyroidism
Constitutional		
Temperature preference	Cool climate	Warm climate
Weight	Loss	Gain
Emotional state	Nervous, easily irritated, highly energetic	Lethargic, complacent, disinterested
Hair	Fine, with hair loss; failure to hold a permanent wave	Coarse, with tendency to break
Skin	Warm, fine, hyperpigmentation at pressure points	Coarse, scaling, dry

HYPERTHYROIDISM VERSUS HYPOTHYROIDISM—cont'd

System or structure Affected	Hyperthyroidism	Hypothyroidism
Fingernails	Thin, with tendency to break; may show oncholysis	Thick
Eyes	Bilateral or unilateral proptosis, lid retraction, double vision	Puffiness in periorbital region
Neck	Goiter, change in shirt neck size, pain over thyroid	No goiter
Cardiac	Tachycardia, arrhythmia, palpitations	No change noted
Gastrointestinal	Increased frequency of bowel movements; diarrhea rare	Constipation
Menstrual	Scant flow, amenorrhea	Menorrhagia
Neuromuscular	Increasing weakness, especially of proximal muscles	Lethargic, but good muscular strength

SAMPLE DOCUMENTATION

Head held erect and midline; features symmetric. Skull reveals no lesions. Male balding pattern with bitemporal loss. No tenderness noted. Scalp moves freely under examining fingers. Temporal arteries palpable but not thickened.

Neck has full range of motion. No torticollis is apparent. Trachea midline; no tug. No lymphadenopathy noted. A 1 × 2 cm nodule is palpated in the right lobe of the thyroid. It is smooth, soft, nontender, and moves freely when patient swallows.

Eyes

EQUIPMENT

- Snellen chart or **E** chart
- Eye cover, gauze, or opaque card
- Rosenbaum or Jaeger near-vision card
- Penlight
- Cotton wisp
- Ophthalmoscope

EXAMINATION

Ask patient to sit or stand.

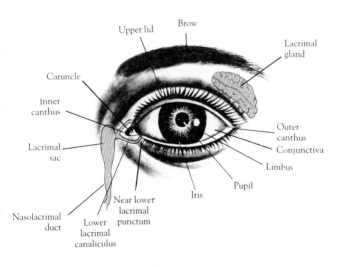

TECHNIQUE	FINDINGS

Visual Testing
Measure visual acuity

♦ Distance vision
Use Snellen test or **E** chart. If tested with and without corrective lenses, test without lenses first and record readings separately.

Expected: Vision 20/20 with or without lenses with near and far vision in each eye. In children:

AGE (YEARS)	ACUITY
3	20/50
4	20/40
5	20/30
6	20/20

Infants: Focus on and track a face or light through 60 degrees.
Unexpected: *Myopia, amblyopia, or presbyopia.*

♦ Near vision
Use near-vision card.
♦ Peripheral vision
Test nasal, temporal, superior, and inferior fields by moving your finger into field from outside.

Unexpected: *Fields of vision more limited than 60 degrees nasally, 90 degrees temporally, 50 degrees superiorly, and 70 degrees inferiorly.*

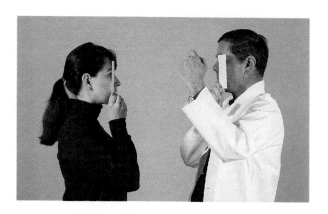

TECHNIQUE	FINDINGS

External Examination
Inspect eyebrows

♦ Size/extension

Expected: Unusually thin if plucked.
Unexpected: End short of temporal canthus.

♦ Hair texture

Unexpected: Coarse.

Inspect orbital area

Unexpected: Edema, puffiness not related to aging, or sagging tissue below orbit. Xanthelasma.

Inspect eyelids

♦ Eyelid position

Unexpected: Ectropion or entropion.

♦ Ability to open wide and close completely
Examine with eyes lightly closed, closed completely, and open wide.

Expected: Superior eyelid covering a portion of iris when open.
Unexpected: Fasciculations when lightly closed. Ptosis. Lagophthalmos.

♦ Eyelid margin

Unexpected: Flakiness, redness, or swelling. Hordeola.

♦ Eyelashes

Expected: Present on both lids. Turned outward.

Palpate eyelids

Unexpected: Nodules.

Palpate the eye

Expected: Can be gently pushed into orbit without discomfort.
Unexpected: Firm and resists palpation.

Pull down lower lids and inspect conjunctivae and sclerae

♦ Color
Inspect upper tarsal conjunctivae only if presence of foreign body is suspected.

Expected: Conjunctivae clear and inapparent. Sclerae white and visible above irides only when eyelids are wide open.

TECHNIQUE	FINDINGS
	Unexpected: Conjunctivae with erythema. Sclerae yellow or green. Sclerae with dark, rust-colored pigment anterior to insertion of medial rectus muscle.
♦ Condition	*Unexpected:* Exudate. Pterygium. Corneal arcus senilis or opacities.

Inspect lacrimal gland region

♦ Lacrimal gland puncta Palpate lower orbital rim near inner canthus. If temporal aspect of upper lid feels full, evert lid and inspect gland.

Expected: Slight elevations with central depression on both upper and lower lid margins.
Unexpected: Enlarged glands. Dry eyes.

Test corneal sensitivity

Touch wisp of cotton to cornea.

Expected: A bilateral blink reflex.

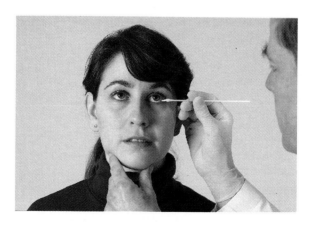

TECHNIQUE	FINDINGS

Inspect external eyes

♦ Corneal clarity
  Shine light tangen-
  tially on cornea

Unexpected: Blood vessels present.

♦ Irides

Expected: Clearly visible pattern.
Similar color.

♦ Pupillary size/shape

Expected: Round, regular, and
equal in size.
*Unexpected: Miosis, mydriasis,
anisocoria, or coloboma.*

♦ Pupillary response to
  light

Expected: Constricting with consensual response of opposite pupil.

♦ Pupillary accommoda-
  tion

Expected: Constricting when
pupils focus on near object or dilat-
ing when focus changes from near
to distant.

Extraocular Eye Muscles
Evaluate muscle balance and movement of eyes

♦ Six cardinal fields of
  gaze
  Hold patient's chin
  and ask patient to
  watch finger or pen-
  light.

Expected: A few horizontal nystag-
mic beats. Smooth, full, coordinated movement of eyes.
*Unexpected: Sustained or jerking
nystagmus. Exposure of sclera from lid
lag.*

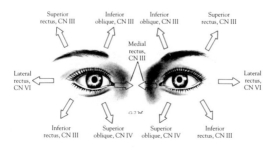

TECHNIQUE	FINDINGS

♦ Corneal light reflex
Direct light to nasal bridge from 30 cm (12 in). Have patient look at nearby object.

Expected: Light reflected symmetrically from both eyes.

♦ Cover-uncover test
Perform if imbalance found with corneal light reflex test. Have patient stare ahead at near, fixed object. Cover one eye and observe other; remove cover and observe uncovered eye. Repeat with other eye.

Unexpected: *Movement of covered or uncovered eye.*

Ophthalmoscopic Examination
Inspect internal eye

♦ Lens clarity
♦ Anterior chamber
Shine focused light tangentially at limbus. Note illumination of iris nasally.

Unexpected: *Shallow chamber. If observed, avoid mydriatics.*

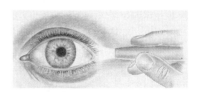

Usual appearance

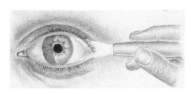

Shallow chamber

TECHNIQUE	FINDINGS

♦ Use the ophthalmo-
scope
With patient looking
at distant object, di-
rect light at pupil from
about 30 cm (12 in).
Move toward patient,
observing:
♦ Red reflex
♦ Fundus

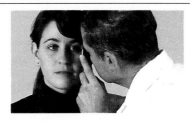

Unexpected: *Opacities.*
Expected: Yellow or pink background, depending on race. Possible crescents or dots at disc margin, usually temporally.
Unexpected: *Discrete areas of
pigmentation away from the disk. Lesions.
Drusen bodies. Hemorrhages.*

♦ Blood vessel charac-
teristics
Follow blood vessels
distally in each quad-
rant noting crossings
of arterioles and
venules.

Expected: Possible venous pulsations (should be documented). A:V
ratio 3:5 or 2:3.
Unexpected: *Glaucomatous cupping,
nicking, crossing, tortuosity.*

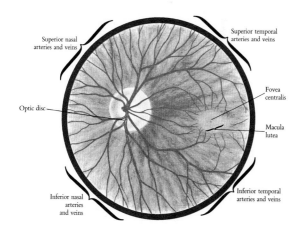

Superior nasal
arteries and veins

Superior temporal
arteries and veins

Fovea
centralis

Optic disc

Macula
lutea

Inferior nasal
arteries
and veins

Inferior temporal
arteries and veins

TECHNIQUE	FINDINGS
◆ Disc characteristics	**Expected:** Yellow to creamy pink, varying by race. Sharp, well-defined margin, especially in temporal region. 1.5 mm diameter. *Unexpected: Myelinated nerve fibers. Papilledema. Glaucomatous cupping.*
◆ Macula densa characteristics Ask patient to look directly at light.	**Expected:** Yellow dot surrounded by deep pink.

AIDS TO DIFFERENTIAL DIAGNOSIS

ABNORMALITY	DESCRIPTION
Strabismus (paralytic and nonparalytic)	Eyes do not focus simultaneously. Can focus separately in nonparalytic type.
Episcleritis	Inflammation of superficial layers of sclera anterior to insertion of rectus muscles. Generally localized with purplish elevation of a few millimeters.
Cataracts	Opacity of lens, generally central, occasionally peripheral.
Diabetic retinopathy (background)	Dot hemorrhages or microaneurysms. Hard exudates (bright yellow, sharply defined borders) and soft exudates (dull yellow spots, poorly defined margins).

SAMPLE DOCUMENTATION

Near vision 20/40 in each eye (OU) without glasses, corrected to 20/20 with glasses. Distant vision 20/20 OU. Visual fields are full to confrontation. Extraocular movements intact and full. No nystagmus. Corneal light reflex equal. Eyebrows are full. No periorbital edema. No ptosis. Conjunctivae are pink and without discharge. Corneal reflex is intact. Anisocoria is present with pupillary size 2 mm OD and 3 mm OS. Pupils react to light directly and consensually and to accommodation. Ophthalmoscopic examination reveals a red reflex. The disc borders are well defined with temporal pigmentation OU. The discs are cream colored. No venous pulsations are noted at the disc. Arteriole-venule ratio is 2:5. No crossing changes are noted. No hemorrhages or exudates are seen. The maculae are yellow OU.

CHAPTER

6
....

Ears, Nose, and Throat

EQUIPMENT

- Otoscope with pneumatic attachment
- Tuning fork
- Nasal speculum
- Tongue blades
- Gloves
- Gauze
- Penlight, sinus transilluminator, or light from otoscope
- Ear specula

EXAMINATION

Have patient sit.

TECHNIQUE	FINDINGS

Ears
Inspect auricles and mastoid area

Examine lateral and medial surfaces and surrounding tissue.

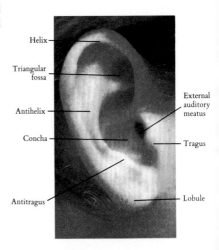

Helix

Triangular fossa

Antihelix

Concha

Antitragus

External auditory meatus

Tragus

Lobule

TECHNIQUE	FINDINGS
♦ Size/shape/symmetry	**Expected:** Familial variations. Auricles of equal size and similar appearance. *Unexpected: Unequal size or configuration. Cauliflower ear and other deformities.*
♦ Landmarks	**Expected:** Darwin tubercle or preauricular pits. *Unexpected: Moles, cysts or other lesions, nodules, or tophi. Openings in preauricular area.*
♦ Color	**Expected:** Same color as facial skin. *Unexpected: Blueness, pallor, or excessive redness.*
♦ Position Draw imaginary line between outer canthus and most prominent protuberance of occiput. Draw imaginary line perpendicular to first line and anterior to auricle.	**Expected:** Top of auricle touching or above line. *Unexpected: Auricle positioned below line; unequal alignment.* **Expected:** Vertical position. *Unexpected: Lateral posterior angle greater than 10 degrees.*
♦ Preauricular area	**Expected:** Skin smooth. *Unexpected: Discharge.*
♦ External auditory canal	**Expected:** No discharge; canal walls pink. *Unexpected: Discharge, purulent, foul smell.*
Palpate auricles and mastoid area	**Expected:** Firm and mobile, readily recoiling from folded position; nontender. *Unexpected: Tenderness, swelling, nodules. Pain from pulling on lobule.*

TECHNIQUE	FINDINGS

Inspect auditory canal with otoscope

Tilt patient's head toward opposite shoulder. Pull auricle upward and back while *gently* inserting speculum. Assess canal from meatus to tympanic membrane. In children, pull auricle downward and back.

Expected: Cerumen in varying color and texture. Pink canal. Hairs in the outer third of the canal.
Unexpected: Cerumen odor, lesions, discharge, scaling, excessive redness, foreign bodies.

Inspect tympanic membrane

♦ Landmarks
Vary light direction to observe entire membrane and annulus.

Expected: Visible umbo, handle of malleus, and light reflex.
Unexpected: Perforations accentuated or not visible.

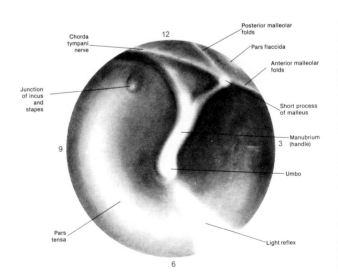

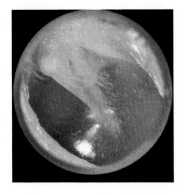

TECHNIQUE	FINDINGS
◆ Color	**Expected:** Translucent, pearly gray. In children, red from crying. *Unexpected: Amber, blue, deep red, chalky white, redness, dullness, white flecks, or dense white plaques.*
◆ Contour	**Expected:** Slightly conical with concavity at umbo. *Unexpected: Bulging (more conical, usually with loss of bony landmarks and distorted light reflex) or retracted (more concave, usually with accentuated bony landmarks and distorted light reflex).*
◆ Mobility Seal canal with speculum, and *gently* apply positive and negative pressure with squeeze bulb.	**Expected:** Movement in and out. In children, tympanic membrane red from crying will be mobile. *Unexpected: No movement.*

Assess hearing

◆ Questions during history	**Expected:** In children, see table on p. 50. *Unexpected: Excessive requests for repetition. Speech with monotonous tone and erratic volume.*

SEQUENCES OF EXPECTED HEARING RESPONSE IN CHILDREN

Age	Response
Birth to 3 months	Startle reflex, crying, cessation of breathing or movement in response to sudden noise; quiets to parent's voice
4 to 6 months	Turns head toward source of sound, but may not always recognize location of sound; responds to parent's voice; enjoys sound-producing toys
6 to 10 months	Responds to own name, telephone ringing, and person's voice, even if not loud; begins localizing sounds above and below, turns head 45 degrees toward sound
10 to 12 months	Recognizes and localizes source of sound; imitates simple words and sounds

TECHNIQUE	FINDINGS
♦ Whispered voice Have patient mask hearing in one ear by moving a finger rapidly up and down in ear canal. Stand 1 to 2 feet from other ear and softly whisper 1 to 2 syllable words. Repeat with untested ear.	**Expected:** Patient repeats words correctly at least 50% of the time. In children, patient should turn toward sound consistently. **Unexpected:** *Patient unable to hear whispered words.*
♦ Ticking watch Have patient mask hearing in one ear. Move watch toward other ear from about 5 inches. Repeat with untested ear.	**Expected:** Patient hears ticking at distance common for most people. **Unexpected:** *Patient unable to hear watch tick.*

INTERPRETATION OF TUNING FORK TESTS

Test	Expected findings	Conductive hearing loss	Sensorineural hearing loss
Weber	No lateralization, but will lateralize to ear occluded by patient	Lateralization to deaf ear unless sensorineural loss	Lateralization to better ear unless conductive loss
Rinne	Air conduction heard longer than bone conduction by 2:1 ratio (*Rinne positive*)	Bone conduction heard longer than air conduction in affected ear (*Rinne negative*)	Air conduction heard longer than bone conduction in affected ear, but less than 2:1 ratio
Schwabach	Examiner hears equally as long as the patient	Patient hears longer than the examiner	Examiner hears longer than the patient

TECHNIQUE	FINDINGS

♦ Weber test
  Place base of vibrating
  tuning fork on midline
  vertex of head. Repeat
  with one ear occluded.

Expected: Sound heard equally in
both ears (unoccluded). Sound
heard better in occluded ear.
Unexpected: See the table on p. 51.

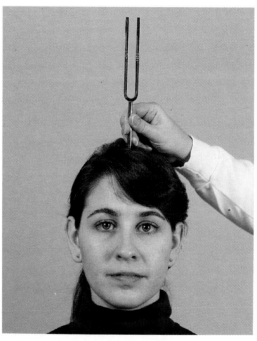

Weber test

♦ Rinne test
  Place base of vibrating
  tuning fork against
  mastoid bone and
  note seconds until
  sound is no longer
  heard, then quickly
  move fork 1 to 2 cm

Expected: Measurement of air-
conducted sound twice as long as
measurement of bone-conducted
sound.
Unexpected: See the table on p. 51.

TECHNIQUE	FINDINGS

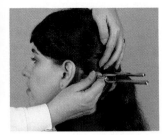 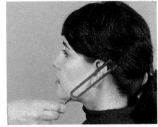

Rinne test

(½ to 1 in) from auditory canal and note seconds until sound is no longer heard. Repeat with other ear.

♦ Schwabach test
Alternately place vibrating tuning fork against patient's mastoid and your mastoid until one of you no longer hears sound.

Expected: Near concurrent loss of sound.
Unexpected: See table on p. 51.

Nose and Sinuses
Inspect external nose

♦ Shape/size

Expected: Smooth. Columella directly midline with width and not greater than diameter of naris.
Unexpected: Swelling or depression of nasal bridge. In children, allergic salute. Transverse crease at junction of nose cartilage and bone.

♦ Color

Expected: Conforms to face color.

♦ Nares

Expected: Oval. Symmetrically positioned.
Unexpected: Asymmetry, discharge, flaring, narrowing.

TECHNIQUE	FINDINGS
Palpate ridge and soft tissues of nose	**Expected:** Firm and stable structures. *Unexpected: Displacement of bone and cartilage, tenderness, or masses.*
Evaluate patency of nares	
Occlude one naris with finger on side of nose and ask patient to breathe through nose. Repeat with other naris.	**Expected:** Noiseless, easy breathing. Newborns: Obligatory nose breathing until 6 months of age. *Unexpected: Noisy breathing; occlusion.*
Inspect nasal mucosa and nasal septum	
Use nasal speculum and strong light. Do not overdilate naris or touch septum.	
♦ Color	**Expected:** Mucosa deep pink and glistening. Turbinates same color as surrounding area. *Unexpected: Increased redness of mucosa or localized redness and swelling in vestibule. Turbinates bluish gray or pale pink.*
♦ Shape	**Expected:** Septum close to midline and fairly straight, thicker anteriorly than posteriorly. Inferior and middle turbinates visible. *Unexpected: Asymmetry of posterior nasal cavities.*

TECHNIQUE	FINDINGS
◆ Condition	**Expected:** Possibly a film of clear discharge on septum. Possibly hairs in vestibule. Turbinates firm. *Unexpected: Discharge, bleeding, crusting, masses, or lesions. Swollen, boggy turbinates. Perforated septum. Polyps.*
Inspect frontal and maxillary sinus area.	*Unexpected: Swelling.*

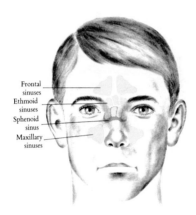

Frontal sinuses
Ethmoid sinuses
Sphenoid sinus
Maxillary sinuses

Palpate frontal and maxillary sinuses

Press thumbs up under bony brow on each side of nose and then under zygomatic processes. Palpate with thumbs or index or middle fingers.	**Expected:** Nontender on palpation. *Unexpected: Tenderness, swelling, or pain.*

TECHNIQUE	FINDINGS

Percuss frontal and maxillary sinuses

Lightly tap with index finger.

Expected: Hollow tone elicited. In children, maxillary sinuses not developed.
Unexpected: Tenderness, swelling, or pain.

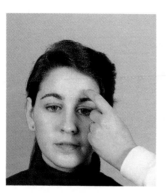 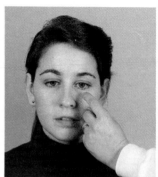

Mouth
Inspect and palpate lips

Have patient remove lipstick (if applicable) and close mouth.

Expected: In infants: sucking calluses, drooling from age 6 weeks to 6 months.
Unexpected: In infants: Drooling persistent after 12 months.

♦ Symmetry

Expected: Symmetric vertically and horizontally at rest and moving.
Unexpected: Asymmetric.

♦ Color

Expected: Pink.
Unexpected: Pallor, circumoral pallor, bluish purple, or cherry red.

♦ Condition

Expected: Smooth.

TECHNIQUE	FINDINGS
	Unexpected: Edema; angioedema; cheilosis; lesions; plaques; vesicles; nodules; ulcerations; or round, oval, or irregular bluish grey macules.

Inspect teeth

♦ Occlusion
Have patient clench teeth and smile with lips spread.

Expected: Upper molars resting directly on lower molars. Upper incisors slightly overriding lower incisors.

Unexpected: Malocclusion.

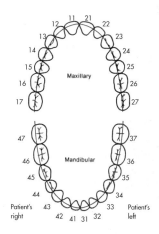

♦ Color

Expected: Ivory.
Unexpected: Stained.

♦ Condition

Expected: 32 teeth. In children, 0 to 20 deciduous teeth until age 6 years. Permanent teeth start erupting around age 6.
Unexpected: Caries and loose or missing teeth.

TECHNIQUE	FINDINGS

Inspect buccal mucosa

Have patient remove
any dental appliances
and then partially
open mouth. Use
tongue blade and
bright light to assess.

♦ Color

Expected: Pinkish red.
Unexpected: Deeply pigmented. Whitish or pinkish scars.

♦ Condition

Expected: Smooth and moist.
Whitish yellow or whitish pink
Stensen duct. Fordyce spots. In infants, nonadherent white patches
(milk).
Unexpected: Red spot at opening of Stensen duct. Round, oval, or irregular bluish gray macules. Ulcers. In infants, adherent white patches.

Inspect and palpate gingiva

Use gloves to palpate.

♦ Color

Expected: Slightly stippled and
pink.
Unexpected: Blue-black line about 1 mm from gum margin.

♦ Condition

Expected: Clearly defined, tight
margin at each tooth. In infants:
Epstein pearls.
Unexpected: Inflammation, swelling, bleeding, lesions, induration, thickening, masses, or tenderness. Enlarged crevices between teeth and gum margins. Pockets containing debris at tooth margins.

Inspect tongue

♦ Size/symmetry

Unexpected: Atrophied.

TECHNIQUE	FINDINGS
◆ Color	**Expected:** Dull red.
◆ Dorsum surface Have patient extend tongue and hold extended.	**Expected:** Moist and glistening. Anterior: smooth yet roughened surface with papillae and small fissures. Posterior: smooth, slightly uneven or rugated surface with thinner mucosa than anterior. Possibly geographic. *Unexpected: Smooth, red, and slick; hairy; swollen; coated; ulcerated; deviation; fasciculations; or limitation of movement.*
◆ Ventral surface and floor of mouth Have patient touch tip of tongue to palate behind upper incisors.	**Expected:** Ventral surface pink and smooth with large veins between frenulum and fimbriated folds. Wharton ducts apparent on each side of frenulum. *Unexpected: Difficulty touching hard palate. Swelling, varicosities.*
◆ Lateral borders Wrap tongue with gauze and pull to each side. Scrape white or red margins to remove food particles.	*Unexpected: Leukoplakia.*

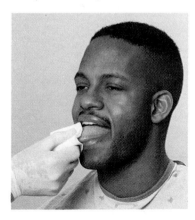

Technique	Findings
Palpate tongue and floor of mouth	Expected: Smooth and even. Unexpected: *Lumps, nodules, induration, ulcerations, or thickened white patches.*

Inspect palate and uvula

Have patient tilt head back.

♦ Color and landmarks

Expected: Hard palate (whitish and dome-shaped with transverse rugae) contiguous with soft palate (pinker than hard). Possible bony protuberance of hard palate at midline (torus palatinus).
Unexpected: *Nodule on palate, not at midline.*

♦ Movement
Ask patient to say, "Ah" while observing soft palate. (Depress tongue if necessary.)

Expected: Soft palate rises symmetrically, with uvula remaining in midline.
Unexpected: *Failure to rise bilaterally. Uvula deviation. Bifid uvula.*

Inspect oropharynx

Depress tongue with tongue blade.

♦ Tonsils

Expected: Tonsils, if present, blend into pink color of pharynx. Possibly crypts in tonsils collecting cellular debris and food particles.
Unexpected: *Tonsils projecting beyond limits of tonsillar pillars. Tonsils red, hypertrophied, and covered with exudate.*

♦ Posterior wall of pharynx

Expected: Smooth, glistening, pink mucosa with some small, irregular spots of lymphatic tissue and small blood vessels.

TECHNIQUE	FINDINGS
	Unexpected: *Red bulge adjacent to tonsil extending beyond midline. Yellowish mucoid film in pharynx. Grayish membrane.*
Elicit gag reflex	
Touch posterior wall of pharynx on each side.	**Expected:** Bilateral response. **Unexpected:** *Unequal response or no response.*

AIDS TO DIFFERENTIAL DIAGNOSIS

ABNORMALITY	DESCRIPTION
Bacterial otitis media	See table on p. 62.
Secretory otitis media (serous otitis media)	See the table on p. 62.
Sinusitis	Fever, headache, local tenderness, pain, swelling of skin overlying involved sinus, and copious purulent nasal discharge.
Tonsillitis	Sore throat, dysphagia, fever, fetid breath, and malaise. Tonsils are red and swollen. Tonsillar crypts filled with purulent exudate. Marked petechial stippling of soft palate. Enlarged tonsillar lymph nodes.
Peritonsillar abscess	Dysphagia, pain radiating to ear, and fever. Tonsil, tonsillar pillar, and adjacent soft palate are red and swollen. Tonsil may appear pushed forward or backward, possibly displacing uvula.
Nasal polyps	Boggy mucosa, rounded, elongated, and extending into nasal cavity.

DIFFERENTIATING BETWEEN OTITIS EXTERNA, BACTERIAL OTITIS MEDIA, AND SECRETORY OTITIS MEDIA

Signs and symptoms	Otitis externa	Bacterial otitis media	Secretory otitis media
Initial symptoms	Itching in ear canal	Fever, feeling of blockage, tugging earlobe	Sticking or cracking sound on yawning or swallowing
Pain	Intense with movement of pinna, chewing	Deep-seated earache	Uncommon; feeling of fullness
Discharge	Watery, then purulent and thick, mixed with pus and epithelial cells; musty, foul-smelling	Only if tympanic membrane ruptures; foul-smelling	Uncommon
Hearing	Conductive loss caused by exudate and swelling of ear canal	Conductive loss as middle ear fills with pus	Conductive loss as middle ear fills with fluid
Inspection	Canal is red, edematous; tympanic membrane obscured	Tympanic membrane is red, thickened, bulging	Tympanic membrane is retracted, yellowish; air bubbles may be present

TECHNIQUE	FINDINGS
Periodontal disease	In mouth with little plaque or calculus, gingivitis with rapid bone and soft tissue degeneration and severe pain.
Malocclusion	Incorrect relationship of positions of teeth of upper and lower jaws.
Dental caries	Discolorations on the crown.
Epiglottitis (children)	High fever, croupy cough, sore throat, drooling; breathing with neck extended.

SAMPLE DOCUMENTATION

Ears. Auricles in alignment, earlobes pierced; no masses, lesions, or tenderness. Canals unobstructed with small amount brown cerumen; tympanic membranes intact, light reflex and bony landmarks present; hearing diminished with bone conduction greater than air conduction with Rinne test and no lateralization with Weber test, unable to repeat whispered words at 1 to 2 feet.

Nose and sinuses. No discharge or polyps, mucosa pink and moist, septum midline, patent bilaterally; no frontal or maxillary tenderness on palpation or percussion.

Mouth and throat. Buccal mucosa pink and moist without lesions; 26 teeth in various states of repair, teeth 25 and 26 missing, 3 loose teeth (33, 34, and 35); gingiva red and boggy; tongue in midline, no lesions or tremors; gag reflex intact, uvula raises evenly; pharynx without redness or exudate; no hoarseness, enunciates words clearly.

CHAPTER

7

....

Chest and Lungs

EQUIPMENT

- ♦ Drape
- ♦ Marking pencil
- ♦ Ruler and tape measure
- ♦ Stethoscope with bell and diaphragm

EXAMINATION

Have patient sit, disrobed to waist.

TECHNIQUE	FINDINGS
Inspect front and back of chest	
See thoracic land-marks.	
♦ Size/shape/symmetry	
♦ Landmarks	**Expected:** Supernumerary nipples possible (but could be clue to other congenital abnormalities).

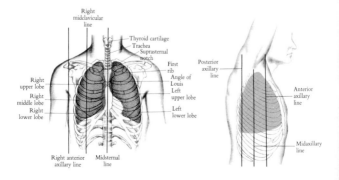

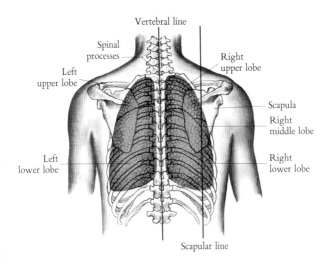

Vertebral line

Spinal
processes

Right
upper lobe

Left
upper lobe

Scapula

Right
middle lobe

Left
lower lobe

Right
lower lobe

Scapular line

TECHNIQUE	FINDINGS
Compare anteroposterior diameter with transverse diameter	**Expected:** Ribs prominent, clavicles prominent superiorly, and sternum usually flat and free of abundance of overlying tissue. Chest somewhat asymmetric. Anterior-posterior diameter often one-half transverse diameter. An infant's chest is expected to measure 2 to 3 cm less than the head circumference.
Unexpected: Barrel chest, posterior or lateral deviation, pigeon chest, or funnel chest.
◆ Assess nails, lips, and nares.	*Unexpected: Clubbed fingernails, pursed lips, flared alae nasi.*
◆ Color
Assess skin, lips, and nails.	*Unexpected: Superficial venous patterns. Cyanosis or pallor of lips or nails.*
◆ Breath	*Unexpected: Malodorous.*

TECHNIQUE	FINDINGS

Evaluate respirations

♦ Rhythm or pattern and rate
See patterns of respiration in the figure below.

Expected: Breathing easy, regular, and without distress. Pattern even. Rate 12-20 respirations/minute. Ratio of respirations to heartbeats about 1:4.

EXPECTED PEDIATRIC RESPIRATIONS

Age	Respirations per minute
Newborn	30-80
1 year	20-40
3 years	20-30
6 years	16-22
10 years	16-20
17 years	12-20

Unexpected: Dyspnea, orthopnea, paroxysmal nocturnal dyspnea, platypnea, tachypnea, and hypopnea. Use of accessory muscles, retractions.

♦ Inspiration/expiration ratio

Unexpected: Air trapping, prolonged expiration.

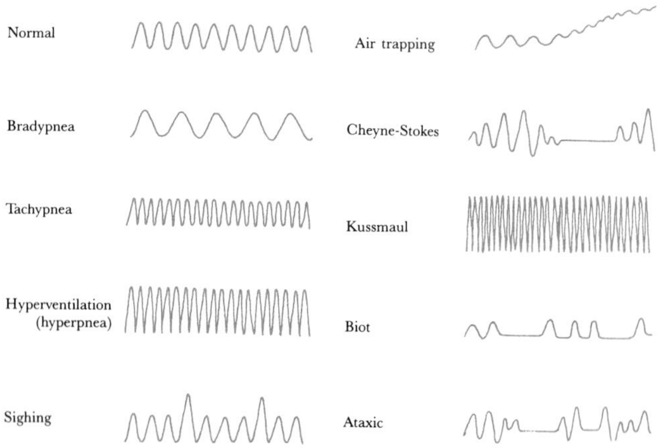

Normal

Bradypnea

Tachypnea

Hyperventilation (hyperpnea)

Sighing

Air trapping

Cheyne-Stokes

Kussmaul

Biot

Ataxic

TECHNIQUE	FINDINGS

**Inspect chest movement
with breathing**

♦ Symmetry

Expected: Chest expansion bilaterally symmetric.
Unexpected: Asymmetry. Unilateral or bilateral bulging. Bulging on expiration.

**Listen to respiration
sounds audible without
stethoscope**

Expected: Generally bronchiovesicular.
Unexpected: Crepitus, stridor, wheezes.

**Palpate thoracic
muscles and skeleton**

♦ Symmetry/condition

Expected: Bilateral symmetry.
Some elasticity of rib cage, but
sternum and xiphoid relatively inflexible and thoracic spine rigid.
*Unexpected: Pulsations, tenderness,
bulges, depressions, unusual movement,
and unusual positions.*

♦ Thoracic expansion
Stand behind patient.
Place palms in light
contact with postero-
lateral surfaces and
thumbs along spinal
processes at tenth rib,
as shown in the figure
at right. Watch thumb
divergence during
quiet and deep
breathing. Face pa-
tient; place thumbs
along costal margin
and xiphoid process
with palms touching
anterolateral chest.
Watch thumb diver-
gence during quiet
and deep breathing.

Expected: Symmetric expansion.
Unexpected: Asymmetric expansion.

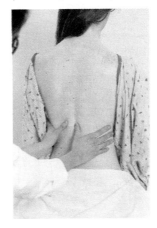

TECHNIQUE	FINDINGS
♦ Sensations	**Expected:** Nontender sensations. *Unexpected: Crepitus or grating vibration.*
♦ Tactile fremitus Ask patient to recite numbers or words while systematically palpating chest with palmer surfaces of fingers or ulnar aspect of clenched fit, using firm, light touch. Assess each area, front to back, side to side, and lung apices. Compare sides.	**Expected:** Great variability. *Unexpected: Decreased or absent fremitus; increased fremitus (coarser, rougher); or gentle, more tremulous fremitus; variation between similar positions on right and left thorax.*

Note position of trachea

Using an index finger or thumbs, palpate gently from suprasternal notch along upper edges of each clavicle and in spaces above, to inner borders of sternocleidomastoid muscles.

Expected: Spaces equal side to side. Trachea midline directly above suprasternal notch. Possible slight deviation to right.
Unexpected: Significant deviation or tug. Pulsations.

Perform direct or indirect percussion on chest

Percuss directly or indirectly, as shown in the top figures on p. 69. Compare all areas bilaterally, following a sequence such as shown in the bottom figures on p. 69. See

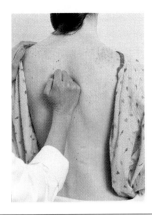
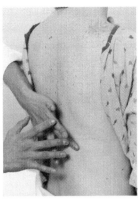

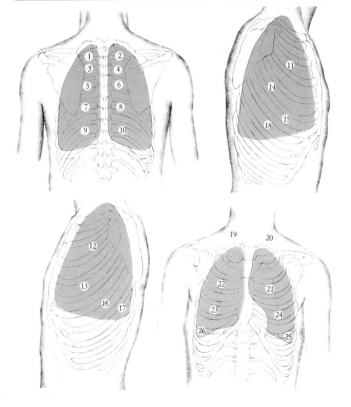

PERCUSSION TONES HEARD OVER THE CHEST

Type of tone	Intensity	Pitch	Duration	Quality
Resonant	Loud	Low	Long	Hollow
Flat	Soft	High	Short	Extremely dull
Dull	Medium	Medium-high	Medium	Thudlike
Tympanic	Loud	High	Medium	Drumlike
Hyper-resonant*	Very loud	Very low	Longer	Booming

From Thompson et al, 1993.
*Hyperresonance is an unexpected sound in adults. It represents air trapping, which occurs in obstructive lung diseases.

TECHNIQUE	FINDINGS
the table above for common tones, intensity, pitch, duration, and quality.	
♦ Thorax	
Have patient sit with head bent and arms folded in front while percussing posterior thorax, then with arms raised overhead while percussing lateral and anterior chest. Percuss at 4 to 5 cm intervals over intercostal spaces, moving superior to inferior, medial to lateral.	**Expected:** Resonance over all areas of lungs, dull over heart and liver, spleen, areas of thorax. Hyperresonance may be heard in children. **Unexpected:** *Hyperresonance, dullness, or flatness.*

TECHNIQUE	**FINDINGS**

♦ Diaphragmatic excursion

Ask patient to breathe deeply and hold breath. Percuss along scapular line on one side until tone changes from resonant to dull. Mark skin. Allow patient to breathe normally, then repeat on other side. Have patient take several breaths, then exhale as much as possible and hold. On each side, percuss up from mark to change from dull to resonant. Tell patient to resume breathing comfortably. Measure excursion distance.

Expected: 3 to 5 cm. Higher on right than left.
Unexpected: Limited descent.

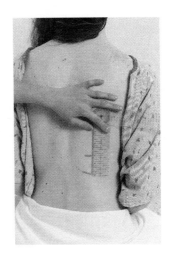

Auscultate chest with stethoscope diaphragm, apex to base

♦ Intensity, pitch, duration, and quality of breath sounds

Have patient breathe slowly and deeply through mouth. Follow set auscultation sequence, holding stethoscope as shown in the figure on p. 72. Ask patient to sit up-

Expected: See expected breath sounds in the table on p. 72. In infants and children, expect transmitted breath sounds throughout the chest. Absent or diminished breath sounds are harder to detect.
Unexpected: Amphoric or cavernous breathing. Sounds difficult to hear or absent. Crackles, rhonchi, wheezes, or pleural friction rub, as described in the table on p. 73.

CHARACTERISTICS OF EXPECTED BREATH SOUNDS

Sound	Characteristics	Findings
Vesicular	Heard over most of lung fields; low pitch; soft and short expirations; will be accentuated in a thin person or a child and diminished in the overweight or very muscular patient	
Bronchovesicular	Heard over main bronchus area and over upper right posterior lung field; medium pitch; expiration equals inspiration	
Bronchial tracheal (tubular)	Heard only over trachea; high pitch; loud and long expirations, often somewhat longer than inspiration	

Modified from Thompson et al, 1993.

TECHNIQUE	FINDINGS
right (1) with head bent and arms folded in front while auscultating posterior thorax, (2) with arms raised overhead while auscultating lateral chest, and (3) with arms down and shoulders back while auscultating anterior chest.	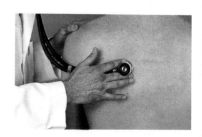

ADVENTITIOUS BREATH SOUNDS

Fine crackles: high-pitched, discrete, discontinuous crackling sounds heard during the end of inspiration; not cleared by cough

Medium crackles: lower, more moist sound heard during the mid-stage of inspiration; not cleared by a cough

Coarse crackles: loud, bubbly noise heard during inspiration; not cleared by a cough

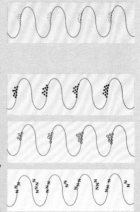

Rhonchi (sonorous wheeze): loud, low, coarse sounds, like a snore, most often heard continuously during inspiration or expiration; coughing may clear sound (usually means mucus accumulation in trachea or large bronchi)

Wheeze (sibilant wheeze): musical noise sounding like a squeak; most often heard continuously during inspiration or expiration; usually louder during expiration

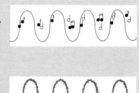

Pleural friction rub: dry, rubbing, or grating sound, usually caused by inflammation of pleural surfaces; heard during inspiration or expiration; loudest over lower lateral anterior surface

Modified from Thompson et al, 1993.

TECHNIQUE	FINDINGS
Listen during inspiration and expiration. Auscultate downward from apex to base at intervals of several centimeters, making side-to-side comparisons.	
♦ Vocal resonance Ask patient to recite numbers or words.	**Expected:** Muffled and indistinct sounds. **Unexpected:** Bronchophony, whispered pectoriloquy, or egophony.

AIDS TO DIFFERENTIAL DIAGNOSIS

ABNORMALITY	SYMPTOM
Lung cancer	Cough, wheezing, emphysema, atelectasis, pneumonitis, and hemoptysis. Possible sputum.
Infections	Sputum production (see the table on p. 75.
Cough-producing conditions	See the box on p. 76.
Asthma	Cough, wheezing, respiratory distress, tachypnea, palor to cyanosis; possible decreased breath sounds; possibly allergy or exercise induced.
Chronic obstructive pulmonary disease	Barrel chest, hyperresonance to percussion, sputum production, cough, prolonged expiration, amphoric breathing.

ASSESSING SPUTUM

Cause	Possible sputum characteristics
Bacterial infection	Yellow, green, rust-colored (blood mixed with yellow sputum), clear, or transparent; purulent; blood streaked; mucoid, viscid
Viral infection	Mucoid, viscid; blood streaked (not common)
Chronic infectious disease	All of the above; particularly abundant in the early morning; slight, intermittent blood streaking; occasionally large amounts of blood
Carcinoma	Slight, persistent blood streaking
Infarction	Blood clotted; large amounts of blood
Tuberculous cavity	Large amounts of blood

SAMPLE DOCUMENTATION

Minimal increase in the anteroposterior diameter of chest, without kyphosis or other distortion. Thoracic expansion symmetric. Respiration rapid and somewhat labored, not accompanied by retractions or stridor. On palpation, trachea in midline without tug; no friction rubs or tenderness over ribs or other bony prominence. Over the left base posteriorly, tactile fremitus is diminished; percussion note was dull; on auscultation, crackles were heard that did not clear with cough; breath sounds diminished. Remainder of lung fields clear and free of adventitious sounds, with resonant percussion tones. On percussion the diaphragm descended 3 cm bilaterally at midscapular line.

Coughs are a common symptom of a respiratory problem. They are usually preceded by a deep inspiration; this is followed by closure of the glottis, relaxation of the diaphragm, and then a sudden, spasmodic expiration, forcing a sudden opening of the glottis. The causes may be related to localized or more general insults at any point in the respiratory tract. Coughs may be voluntary, but they are usually reflexive responses to an irritant such as a foreign body (microscopic or larger), an infectious agent, or a mass of any sort compressing the respiratory tree. They may also be a clue to an anxiety state.

Describe a cough according to its moisture, frequency, regularity, pitch and loudness, and quality. The type of cough may offer some clue to the cause. Although a cough may not have a serious cause, it should not be ignored.

Dry or moist. A moist cough may be caused by infection and can be accompanied by sputum production. A dry cough can have a variety of causes (for example, cardiac problems, allergies, or AIDS), which may be indicated by the quality of its sound.

Onset. An acute onset, particularly with fever, suggests infection; in the absence of fever, a foreign body or inhaled irritants are additional possible causes.

Frequency of occurrence. Note whether the cough is seldom or often present. An infrequent cough may result from allergens or environmental insults.

Regularity. A regular, paroxysmal cough is heard in pertussis. An irregularly occurring cough may have a variety of causes, such as smoking, early congestive heart failure, an inspired foreign body or irritant, or a tumor within or compressing the bronchial tree.

Pitch and loudness. A cough may be loud and high pitched or quiet and relatively low pitched.

Postural influences. A cough may occur soon after a person has reclined or assumed an erect position (for example, with a nasal drip or pooling of secretions in the upper airway).

Quality. A dry cough may sound brassy if it is caused by compression of the respiratory tree (as by a tumor) or hoarse if it is caused by croup. Pertussis produces an inspiratory "whoop" at the end of a paroxysm of coughing.

CHAPTER

8
....

Heart and Blood Vessels

EQUIPMENT
- ♦ Tangential light source
- ♦ Marking pencil
- ♦ Stethoscope with bell and diaphragm
- ♦ Sphygmomanometer
- ♦ Centimeter ruler

EXAMINATION

TECHNIQUE	FINDINGS

Heart

Inspect precordium

Have patient supine
and keep the light
source tangential

♦ Apical impulse

Expected: Visible about midclavicular line in fifth left intercostal space. Sometimes only visible with patient sitting.
Unexpected: *Readily visible and palpable with supine patient; visible in more than one intercostal space; absence of impulse, in addition to faint heart sounds, particularly in left lateral recumbent position; or exaggerated lifts or heaves.*

TECHNIQUE	FINDINGS

Palpate precordium and carotid artery

♦ Apical impulse
Have patient supine.
With hands *warm*,
gently feel pre-
cordium, using proxi-
mal halves of the fin-
gers held together or
whole hand. As shown
in the figure at right,
methodically move
from apex to left ster-
nal border, base, right
sternal border, epigas-
trium, and axillae.

Expected: Gentle, brief impulse,
palpable within radius of 1 cm or
less, although often not felt.
Unexpected: *Heave or lift, loss of thrust,
displacement to right or left; or thrill.*

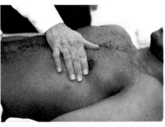

♦ Carotid artery
Use other hand to
palpate carotid artery,
as shown in the figure
at right, to describe
carotid pulse in rela-
tion to cardiac cycle.
Locate each sensation
in terms of its inter-
costal space and rela-
tionship to midster-
nal, midclavicular, and
axillary lines.

Expected: Carotid pulse and first
heart sound (S_1) practically syn-
chronous.
Unexpected: *Asynchrony.*

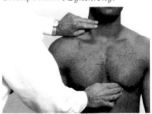

Percuss precordium (optional)

Begin by tapping at
anterior axillary line,
moving medially along
intercostal spaces to-
ward sternal borders
until tone changes
from resonance to
dullness. Mark skin
with pencil.

Expected: No change in tone before right sternal border; on left,
loss of resonance generally close to
point of maximal impulse at fifth
intercostal space. Loss of resonance may outline the left border
of heart at second to fifth intercostal spaces.

TECHNIQUE	FINDINGS

Auscultate in the five auscultatory areas

Make certain patient is warm and relaxed. Isolate each sound and each pause in the cycle, and then inch along with the stethoscope. Approach each of the five precordial areas shown in the figure below systematically, base to apex or apex to base, using each of the positions shown in the figures at right. Use the diaphragm of the stethoscope first, with firm pressure, then the bell, with light pressure.

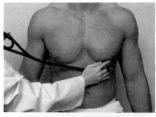

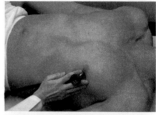

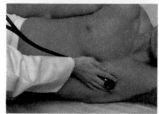

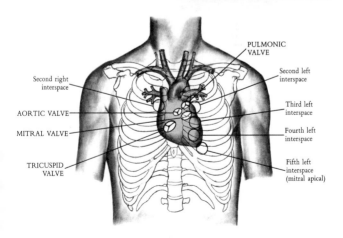

PULMONIC VALVE

Second left interspace

Second right interspace

AORTIC VALVE

MITRAL VALVE

TRICUSPID VALVE

Third left interspace

Fourth left interspace

Fifth left interspace (mitral apical)

HEART SOUNDS ACCORDING TO AUSCULTATORY AREA

	Aortic	Pulmonic	Second pulmonic	Mitral	Tricuspid
Pitch	$S_1 < S_2$	$S_1 < S_2$	$S_1 < S_2$	$S_1 < S_2$	$S_1 < S_2$
Loudness	$S_1 < S_2$	$S_1 < S_2$	$S_1 < S_2$*	$S_1 > S_2$†	$S_1 > S_2$
Duration	$S_1 > S_2$	$S_1 > S_2$	$S_1 > S_2$	$S_1 > S_2$	$S_1 > S_2$
S_2 split	>Inhale <Exhale	>Inhale <Exhale	>Inhale <Exhale	>Inhale‡ <Exhale	>Inhale <Exhale
A_2	Loudest	Loud	Decreased		
P_2	Decreased	Louder	Loudest		

*S_1 is relatively louder in second pulmonic area than in aortic area.
†S_1 may be louder in mitral area than in tricuspid area.
‡S_2 split may not be audible in mitral area if P_2 is inaudible.

TECHNIQUE	FINDINGS
♦ Rate and rhythm Assess overall rate and rhythm.	**Expected:** Rate 60 to 90/minutes, regular rhythm. **Unexpected:** *Bradycardia, tachycardia,* *dysrhythmia.*
♦ S_1 Ask patient to breathe comfortably, then hold breath in expiration. Listen for S_1 (best heard toward apex) while palpating carotid pulse. Note in- tensity, variations, ef- fect of respiration, and splitting. Concentrate on systole, then dias- tole.	**Expected:** S_1 usually heard as one sound and coincides with rise of carotid pulse. See the table on p. 80 and the figure below. **Unexpected:** *Extra sounds or murmurs.*

HEART SOUNDS		AREA BEST HEARD
S_1 S_2	Intense first sound	Apex
S_1 M T S_2	Split first sound	Tricuspid
S_1 S_2	Intense second sound	Base
S_1 S_2 S_1 S_2 A P	Physiological splitting—S_2 Expiration Inspiration	Base
S_1 S_2 S_3	Third sound (ventricular gallop)	Apex
S_4 S_1 S_2	Fourth sound (atrial gallop)	Apex
S_1 S_2 S_{3-4}	Summation gallop	Apex

EXTRA HEART SOUNDS

Sound	Detection	Description
Increased S_3	Bell at apex; patient left lateral recumbent	Early diastole, low pitch
Increased S_4	Bell at apex; patient supine or semilateral	Late diastole or early systole, low pitch
Gallops	Bell at apex; patient supine or left lateral recumbent	Presystole, intense, easily heard
Mitral valve opening snap	Diaphragm medial to apex, may radiate to base; any position, second left intercostal	Early diastole briefly, before S_3; high pitch, sharp snap or click; not affected by respiration; easily confused with S_2
Ejection clicks	Diaphragm; patient sitting or supine	
Aortic valve	Apex, base in second right intercostal space	Early systole, intense, high pitch; radiates; not affected by respirations
Pulmonary valve	Second left intercostal space at sternal border	Early systole, less intense than aortic click; intensifies on expiration, decreases on inspiration
Pericardial friction rub	Widely heard, sound clearest toward apex	May occupy all of systole and diastole; intense, grating, machinelike; may have three components and obliterate heart sounds; if only one or two components, may sound like murmur

TECHNIQUE	FINDINGS
♦ S$_2$ Ask patient to breathe comfortably as you listen for S$_2$ (best heard in aortic and pulmonic areas) to become two components during inspiration. Ask patient to inhale and hold breath.	**Expected:** S$_2$ to become two components during inspiration. S$_2$ to become an apparent single sound as breath exhaled. See the table on p. 80 and the figure on p. 81.
♦ Splitting	**Expected:** S$_2$ splitting—greatest at peak of inspiration—varying from easily heard to nondetectable.
♦ S$_3$ and S$_4$ If needed, ask patient to raise a leg to increase venous return or to grip your hand vigorously and repeatedly to increase arterial pressure.	**Expected:** Both S$_3$ and S$_4$ quiet and difficult to hear. **Unexpected:** *Increased intensity (and ease of hearing) of either.*
♦ Extra heart sounds	**Unexpected:** *Extra heart sounds—snaps, clicks, friction rubs, and murmurs. See the table on p. 82 and the figure on p. 81.*
Assess characteristics of murmurs	
♦ Timing and duration, pitch, intensity, pattern, quality, location, radiation, respiratory phase variations	See the table on p. 82. In children it is necessary to distinguish innocent murmurs from organic murmurs caused by congenital defect or rheumatic fever.

TECHNIQUE	FINDINGS

Peripheral Arteries
Palpate arterial pulses in distal extremities

Palpate carotid, brachial, radial, femoral, popliteal, dorsalis pedis, and posterior tibial arteries, using distal pads of second and third fingers, as shown in the figure on p. 85.

♦ Characteristics
Compare characteristics bilaterally, as well as between upper and lower extremities.

Expected: Femoral pulse as strong as or stronger than radial pulse.
Unexpected: Femoral pulse weaker than radial pulse or absent, alternating pulse (pulsus alternans), pulsus bisferiens, bigeminal pulse (pulsus bigeminus), bounding pulse, labile pulse, paradoxic pulse (pulsus paradoxus), pulsus differens, tachycardia, trigeminal pulse (pulsus trigeminus), or water-hammer pulse (Corrigan pulse).

♦ Rate

Expected: 60 to 90/minute.

PEDIATRIC HEART RATE

AGE	BEATS PER MINUTE
Newborn	120-170
1 year	80-160
3 years	80-120
6 years	75-115
10 years	70-110

♦ Rhythm

Expected: Regular.
Unexpected: Irregular, either in a pattern or patternless.

♦ Contour

Expected: Smooth, rounded, or domed shape.

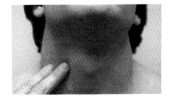

Carotid

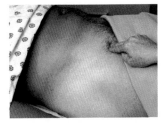

Brachial

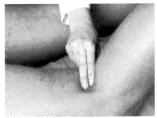

Radial

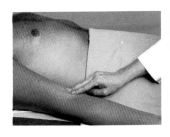

Femoral

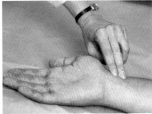

Popliteal

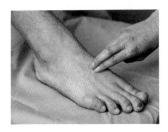

Dorsalis pedis

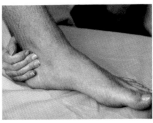

Posterior tibial

TECHNIQUE	FINDINGS
♦ Amplitude	*Unexpected:* Bounding, full, diminished, or absent. Describe on scale of 0 to 4: 4 = bounding 3 = full, increased 2 = expected 1 = diminished 0 = absent, not palpable

Auscultate carotid, temporal, abdominal aorta, renal, and femoral, and iliac arteries for bruits

You may at times need to ask patient to hold breath for a few heartbeats and auscultate with bell of stethoscope.

Unexpected: Transmitted murmurs, vigorous left ventricular ejection, obstruction in cervical arteries. In children it is not unusual to hear a venous hum over internal jugular veins. There is usually no pathologic significance.

Assess for arterial occlusion and insufficiency

♦ Site
Assess for pain distal to possible occlusion.

Unexpected: Dull ache accompanied by fatigue and often crampiness; possible constant or excruciating pain. Weak, thready, or absent pulses; systolic bruits over arteries; loss of body warmth; localized pallor or cyanosis; delay in venous filling; or thin, atrophied skin, muscle atrophy, and loss of hair.

♦ Degree of occlusion
Ask patient to lie supine. Elevate extremity and note de-

Expected: Slight pallor on elevation and return to full color as soon as leg becomes dependent.

TECHNIQUE	FINDINGS
gree of blanching, then ask patient to sit on edge of table or bed to lower extremity. Note time for maximal return of color when extremity is elevated.	*Unexpected:* *Delay of more than 2 seconds.*

Measure blood pressure

Measure in both arms at least once. Patient's arm should be slightly flexed and comfortably supported on table, pillow, or your hand. When measuring an infant's blood pressure, use the flush technique if needed.

Expected: 100 to 140 mm Hg systolic and 60 to 90 mm Hg second diastolic, with pulse pressure of 30 to 40 mm Hg (sometimes to 50 mm Hg). Reading between arms may vary by as much as 10 mm Hg; usually higher in right arm.
Unexpected: *Hypertension (see the table on p. 88).*

Peripheral Veins
Assess jugular venous pressure

Ask patient to recline at 45-degree angle. With tangential light, observe both jugular veins. As shown in the figure at right, use a centimeter ruler to measure vertical distance between angle of Louis (manubriosternal joint) and highest level of jugular vein pulsation on both sides.

Expected: Pressure of 2 cm or less, bilaterally symmetric.
Unexpected: *Abnormal distention or distention on one side.*

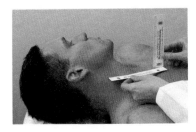

CLASSIFICATION OF HYPERTENSION BY AGE-GROUP

Age-group	Significant hyper-tension (mm Hg)	Severe hyper-tension (mm Hg)
Newborn		
7 days	Systolic BP ≥ 96	Systolic BP ≥ 106
8-30 days	Systolic BP ≥ 104	Systolic BP ≥ 110
Infant (<2 yr)	Systolic BP ≥ 112	Systolic BP ≥ 118
	Diastolic BP ≥ 74	Diastolic BP ≥ 82
Child		
(3-5 yr)	Systolic BP ≥ 116	Systolic BP ≥ 124
	Diastolic BP ≥ 76	Diastolic BP ≥ 84
(6-9 yr)	Systolic BP ≥ 122	Systolic BP ≥ 130
	Diastolic BP ≥ 78	Diastolic BP ≥ 86
(10-12 yr)	Systolic BP ≥ 126	Systolic BP ≥ 134
	Diastolic BP ≥ 82	Diastolic BP ≥ 90
Adolescent		
(13-15 yr)	Systolic BP ≥ 136	Systolic BP ≥ 144
	Diastolic BP ≥ 86	Diastolic BP ≥ 92
(16-18 yr)	Systolic BP ≥ 142	Systolic BP ≥ 150
	Diastolic BP ≥ 92	Diastolic BP ≥ 98
Adult	Systolic BP ≥ 160	Systolic BP ≥ 240
	Diastolic BP ≥ 90	Diastolic BP ≥ 115

Calculation of systolic blood pressure expected for children over 1 year can be estimated with the following formula:

$$80 + (2 \times \text{child's age in years})$$

For example, the calculation of the expected systolic blood pressure of a 5-year-old would be as follows:

$$80 + (2 \times 5) = 90$$

Although this calculation gives a figure below the expected mean, it is still considered within normal limits for a 5-year-old child.

Modified from National Heart, Lung, and Blood Institute, 1987. Used with permission.

TECHNIQUE	FINDINGS

**Assess for venous
obstruction and
insufficiency**

Inspect extremities,
with patient both
standing and supine.

♦ Affected area

Unexpected: *Constant pain with
swelling and tenderness over muscles,
engorgement of superficial veins, and
cyanosis.*

♦ Thrombosis
Flex patient's knee
slightly with one hand
and with other, dorsi-
flex foot to test for
Homans sign.

Unexpected: *Redness, thickening, and
tenderness along superficial vein. Calf
pain with test for Homans sign.*

♦ Edema
Press index finger over
bony prominence of
tibia or medial malle-
olus for several sec-
onds.

Unexpected: *Orthostatic (pitting)
edema; thickening and ulceration of skin
possible. Grade edema 1+ to 4+ as
follows:*

*1+ = Slight pitting, no visible distortion,
disappears rapidly*

*2+ = Deeper than 1+ and disappears in
10 to 15 seconds*

*3+ = Noticeably deep and may last more
than 1 minute, with dependent extremity
full and swollen*

*4+ = Very deep and lasts 2 to 5 minutes,
with grossly distorted dependent extremity*

♦ Varicose veins
If suspected, have pa-
tient stand on toes 10
times in succession.

Expected: Pressure from toe
standing disappears in seconds.
Unexpected: *Veins dilated and swollen;
often tortuous when extremities are
dependent and pressure does not quickly
disappear.*

TECHNIQUE	FINDINGS
If varicose veins are present, assess venous incompetence with Trendelenburg test: ask patient to lie supine, lift leg above heart level until veins empty, then quickly lower leg.	**Unexpected:** *Rapid filling of veins.*
Evaluate patency of deep veins with Perthes test: Ask patient to lie supine. Elevate extremity and occlude subcutaneous veins with tourniquet just above knee. Then ask patient to walk.	**Unexpected:** *Superficial veins fail to empty.*
Evaluate direction of blood flow and presence of compensatory circulation: Put affected limb in dependent position, then empty or strip vein. Release pressure of one finger to assess blood flow; if necessary, repeat and release pressure of other finger.	**Unexpected:** *Stripped vessel fills before pressure is released, or blood does not refill vein when pressure is released.*

AIDS TO DIFFERENTIAL DIAGNOSIS

ABNORMALITY	DESCRIPTION
Chest pain	See the box on p. 91.
Left ventricular hypertrophy	Vigorous sustained lift palpable during ventricular systole, sometimes over broader area than usual (by 2 cm or more).

CHEST PAIN

Type of chest pain	Characteristics
Anginal	Substernal; provoked by effort, emotion, eating; relieved by rest and/or nitroglycerin
Pleural	Precipitated by breathing or coughing; usually described as sharp
Esophageal	Burning, substernal, occasional radiation to the shoulder; nocturnal occurrence, usually when lying flat; relief with food, antacids, sometimes nitroglycerin
From a peptic ulcer	Almost always infradiaphragmatic and epigastric; nocturnal occurrence and daytime attacks relieved by food; unrelated to activity
Biliary	Usually under right scapula, prolonged in duration; will trigger angina more often than mimic it
Arthritic/ bursitis	Usually of hours-long duration; local tenderness and/or pain with movement
Cervical	Associated with injury; provoked by activity, persists after activity; painful on palpation and/or movement
Musculo skeletal (chest)	Intensified or provoked by movement, particularly twisting or costochondral bending; long lasting; often associated with local tenderness
Psychoneurotic	Associated with/after anxiety; poorly described; located in intramammary region

Unlike in adults, chest pain in children and adolescents is seldom caused by a cardiac problem. It is very often difficult to find a cause, but trauma and exercise-induced asthma and the use of cocaine, even in a somewhat younger child as in the adolescent and adult, should be among the considerations.

Modified from Samly, 1987; Harvey, 1988.

ABNORMALITY	DESCRIPTION
	Displacement of apical impulse can be well lateral to midclavicular line and downward.
Right ventricular hypertrophy	Lift along left sternal border in third and fourth left intercostal spaces accompanied by occasional systolic retraction at apex. Left ventricle displaced and turned posteriorly by enlarged right ventricle.
Congestive heart failure	Congestion in pulmonary or systemic circulation. Can be predominantly left- or right-sided and can develop gradually or suddenly with acute pulmonary edema.
Cor pulmonale	Left parasternal systolic lift and loud S_2.
Myocardial infarction	Deep substernal or visceral pain, often radiating to jaw, neck, and left arm (although discomfort is sometimes mild); dysrhythmias; S_4 usually present; heart sounds distant, with soft, systolic, blowing murmur; pulse possibly thready; varied blood pressure (although hypertension usual in early phases).
Myocarditis	Initial: fatigue, dyspnea, fever, and palpitations. Later: cardiac enlargement, murmur, gallop rhythms, tachycardia, dysrhythmias, and pulsus alternans.
Conduction disturbances	Transient weakness, fainting spells, or strokelike episodes.

ABNORMALITY	DESCRIPTION
Congenital defects	
Tetralogy of Fallot	Parasternal heave and precordial prominence. Cyanosis. Systolic ejection murmur heard over third intercostal space, sometimes radiating to left side of neck. Single S_2.
Ventricular septal defect	Arterial pulse small, and jugular venous pulse unaffected. Regurgitation occurs through septal defect, resulting in holosystolic murmur that is frequently loud, coarse, high-pitched, and best heard along the left sternal border in the third to fifth intercostal spaces. Distinct lift often discernible along left sternal border and the apical area. Does not radiate to neck.
Coarctation of the aorta	Delay and/or palpable diminution in amplitude (not necessarily an absence) of femoral pulse when radial and femoral pulses are palpated simultaneously. Findings are same on right and left sides. Blood pressure in arms will be distinctly, even severely, higher than in legs. Possible systolic murmur audible over precordium and sometimes over back relative to area of coarctation. Adult x-ray examination may show notching of ribs and "3" sign in contour of left upper border of heart.

ABNORMALITY	DESCRIPTION
Patent ductus arteriosus	Neck vessels dilated and pulsate, and pulse pressure wide. Harsh, loud, continuous murmur with machinelike quality, heard at first to third intercostal spaces and lower sternal border. Murmur usually unaltered by postural change.
Atrial septal defect	Systolic ejection murmur—best heard over pulmonic area—that is diamond shaped, often loud, high in pitch, and harsh. May be accompanied by brief, rumbling, early diastolic murmur. Does not usually radiate beyond precordium. Systolic thrill may be felt over area of murmur along with palpable parasternal thrust. S_2 may be split fairly widely. Particularly significant with palpable thrust and occasional radiation through to back.
Dextrocardia and situs inversus	Altered clinical manifestations of disease (e.g., the substernal pressure of myocardial ischemia may be felt to the right of the precordium and may more often radiate to right arm).

Arterial/venous disorders

Arterial aneurysm	Pulsatile swelling along course of an artery—most commonly in the aorta, although abdominal, renal, femoral, and popliteal arteries

ABNORMALITY	DESCRIPTION
	are also common. Thrill or bruit sometimes evident over aneurysm.
Venous thrombosis	Clinical findings in superficial vein include redness, thickening, and tenderness along involved segment. Deep vein thrombosis in femoral and pelvic circulations may be asymptomatic, but suggestive signs and symptoms include tenderness along iliac vessels and femoral canal, in popliteal space, and over deep calf veins, as well as slight swelling, minimal ankle edema, low-grade fever, and tachycardia.
Raynaud disease	Intermittent skin pallor or cyanosis, bilateral and lasting from minutes to hours. Skin over digits eventually appears smooth, shiny, and tight; ulcers may appear on tips of digits.
Mitral insufficiency	Usually silent and painless. Also occurs after infarction.
Atherosclerotic heart disease	Myocardial insufficiency, angina pectoris, dysrhythmias, and congestive heart failure.
Angina	Substernal pain or intense pressure radiating at times to neck, jaws, and arms, particularly the left arm. Often accompanied by shortness of breath, fatigue, diaphoresis, faintness, and syncope.

SAMPLE DOCUMENTATION

Apical impulse in otherwise quiet precordium palpated in fifth left intercostal space at midclavicular line. No lifts, heaves, or thrills felt on palpation. S_1 and S_2 not exaggerated or diminished; physiologic splitting of S_2; S_3 and S_4 not heard. Grade I/VI midsystolic (ejection) murmur heard at base in second left intercostal space, sharply localized. Peripheral vascular: pulses easily palpated over radials, carotids, femorals, posterior tibials, and dorsalis pedis; equal, regular, rate of 78/min. Blood pressure 136/86/72 right arm, 140/86/72 left arm, sitting. No edema or varicose veins in lower extremities.

9

Breasts and Axillae

EQUIPMENT

♦ Ruler (if mass detected)
♦ Flashlight with transilluminator (if mass detected)
♦ Glass slide and cytologic fixative (for nipple discharge)
♦ Small pillow or folded towel

EXAMINATION

TECHNIQUE	FINDINGS

Females

With patient seated and arms hanging loosely, inspect both breasts

Inspect all quadrants and tail of Spence as shown in the figure. If necessary, lift breasts with fingertips to expose lower and lateral aspects.

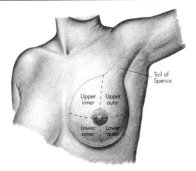

♦ Size/shape/symmetry

Expected: Convex, pendulous, or conical. Frequently asymmetric in size.

♦ Texture/contour

Expected: Smooth and uninterrupted.
Unexpected: *Dimpling or peau d'orange appearance. Changes or asymmetric appearance.*

♦ Skin color

Expected: Consistent color.
Unexpected: *Areas of discoloration or asymmetric appearance.*

TECHNIQUE	FINDINGS
◆ Venous patterns	**Expected:** Bilateral venous networks, although pronounced generally only in pregnant or obese women. *Unexpected: Unilateral network.*
◆ Markings	**Expected:** Long-standing nevi. Supernumerary nipples possible (but could be a clue to other congenital abnormalities). *Unexpected: Changing or tender nevi. Lesions.*

Inspect areolae and nipples

◆ Size/shape/symmetry	**Expected:** Areola round or oval, bilaterally equal or nearly equal. Nipples bilaterally equal or nearly equal in size and usually everted, although one or both sometimes inverted. *Unexpected: Recent unilateral nipple inversion or retraction.*
◆ Color	**Expected:** Areolae and nipples pink to brown. *Unexpected: Nonhomogeneous in color.*
◆ Texture/contour	**Expected:** Areolae smooth, except for Montgomery tubercles. Nipples smooth or wrinkled. *Unexpected: Areola with suppurative or tender Montgomery tubercles or with peau d'orange appearance. Nipples crusting, cracking, or with discharge.*

With patient in the following positions, reinspect both breasts

◆ Arms extended over head	**Expected, all positions:** Breasts bilaterally equal with even contour.

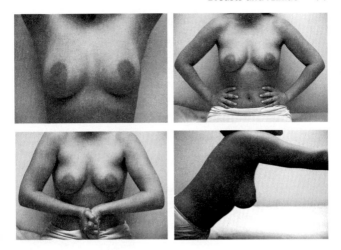

TECHNIQUE	FINDINGS
◆ Hands pressed on hips or pushed together in front of chest ◆ Seated and leaning over ◆ Recumbent	*Unexpected:* *Dimpling, retraction, deviation, or fixation of breasts.*
With patient seated and arms hanging loosely, palpate breasts	
First palpate entire breast lightly, then repeat with deeper, heavier palpation. Using finger pads, systematically palpate both breasts in all four quadrants and over	Expected: Tissue generally dense, firm, and elastic, but sometimes lobular. The inframammary ridge may be felt along lower edge of breast. During menstrual cycle, cyclic pattern of breast enlargement, increased nodularity, and tenderness.

TECHNIQUE	FINDINGS
the areola. Push gently but firmly toward chest while rotating fingers clockwise or counterclockwise, following a *back-and-forth*, *concentric circle*, or *wedge* pattern.	*Unexpected:* Lumps or nodules. Characterize any masses by location, size, shape, consistency, tenderness, mobility, delineation of borders, and retraction. Use transillumination to assess presence of fluid in masses.

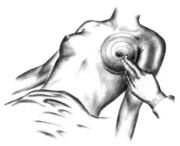 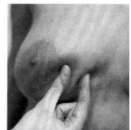

For large breasts, perform bimanual palpation, immobilizing inferior surface with one hand while examining superior surface with the other hand.

With patient seated and arms raised over her head, palpate tail of Spence

Gently compress tissue between thumb and fingers.	**Expected:** Similar to expected findings on p. 99, with patient's arms hanging loosely.
	Unexpected: Similar to unexpected findings above with patient's arms hanging loosely.

TECHNIQUE	FINDINGS

With patient seated and arms flexed at the elbows, palpate for lymph nodes.

Left side: Support patient's lower left arm with your left hand while examining the left axilla with your right hand. With palmar surface of fingers, reach deep into hollow, pushing firmly upward, then bring fingers down, gently rolling soft tissue against chest wall and axilla. Explore apex, medial, and lateral aspects along rib cage; lateral aspects along upper surface of arm; and anterior and posterior walls of axilla. Hook fingers over clavicle and rotate over supraclavicular area while patient turns head toward same side and raises shoulder.
Repeat on right side.

Unexpected: *Nodes, especially in supraclavicular area. Describe nodes by location, size, shape, consistency, tenderness, fixation, and delineation of borders.*

TECHNIQUE	FINDINGS

Palpate and compress nipples

Gently compress between thumb and index finger as shown.

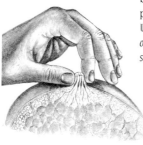

Expected: Possible nipple erection and areola puckering. Breast enlargement is not unusual in newborns. "Witch's milk" may be expressed.
Unexpected: Discharge. *Note color and origin of any discharge and prepare smear.*

With patient supine, continue palpation of breast tissue

Have patient put one hand behind head. Place a towel under shoulder of same side. Compress breast tissue between fingers and chest wall, using rotary motion of fingers. Have patient place arm at her side, and repeat palpation. Repeat with other breast.

Expected: Similar to expectations of patient seated, with arms hanging loosely.
Unexpected: *Similar to unexpected findings of patient seated, with arms hanging loosely.*

Males
Inspect both breasts

♦ Size/shape/symmetry
♦ Surface characteristics

Expected: Even with chest wall. Sometimes convex (especially overweight men).
Unexpected: *Enlarged breasts.*

TECHNIQUE	FINDINGS

**Inspect areolae
and nipples**

♦ Size/shape/symmetry

Expected: Areola round or oval, bilaterally equal or nearly equal. Nipples bilaterally equal or nearly
equal in size and usually everted,
although one or both sometimes
inverted.
*Unexpected: Recent unilateral nipple
inversion or retraction.*

♦ Color

Expected: Areolae and nipples
pink to brown.
Unexpected: Nonhomogeneous in color.

♦ Texture/contour

Expected: Areolae smooth, except
for Montgomery tubercles. Nipples
smooth or wrinkled.
*Unexpected: Areolae with suppurative or
tender Montgomery tubercles or with peau
d'orange appearance. Nipples crusting,
cracking, or with discharge.*

**Palpate breasts and
over areolae**

Palpate briefly, follow-
ing palpation steps for
"Females."

Expected: Thin layer of fatty tissue
overlying muscle. Thick layer in
obese men may give appearance of
breast enlargement. Firm disk of
glandular tissue sometimes evi-
dent.
Unexpected: Lumps or nodules.

**With patient seated and
arms flexed at the
elbows, palpate for
lymph nodes**

Left side: Support pa-
tient's lower left arm
with your left hand

*Unexpected: Nodes, especially in
supraclavicular area. Describe nodes by
location, size, shape, consistency,*

TECHNIQUE	FINDINGS
while examining left axilla with your right hand. With palmar surface of fingers, reach deep into hollow, pushing firmly upward, then bring fingers down, gently rolling soft tissue against chest wall and axilla. Explore apex, medial, and lateral aspects along rib cage; lateral aspects along upper surface of arm; and anterior and posterior walls of axilla. Hook fingers over clavicle and rotate over supraclavicular area while patient turns head toward same side and raises shoulder. Repeat on right side.	*tenderness, fixation, and delineation of borders.*

Palpate and compress nipples

Gently compress between thumb and index finger.	**Expected:** Possible nipple erection and areola puckering. Breast enlargement is not unusual in newborns. "Witch's milk" may be expressed. **Unexpected:** Discharge. *Note color and origin of any discharge and prepare smear.*

DIFFERENTIATING SIGNS AND SYMPTOMS OF BREAST MASSES

	Fibrocystic disease	Fibroadenoma	Cancer
Age	20-49	15-55	30-80
Occurrence	Usually bilateral	Usually bilateral	Usually unilateral
Number	Multiple or single	Single; may be multiple	Single
Shape	Round	Round or discoid	Irregular or stellate
Consistency	Soft to firm; tense	Firm, rubbery	Hard, stonelike
Mobility	Mobile	Mobile	Fixed
Retraction signs	Absent	Absent	Often present
Tenderness	Usually tender	Usually nontender	Usually nontender
Delimitation	Well delineated	Well delineated	Poorly delineated; irregular
Variation with menses	Yes	No	No

AIDS TO DIFFERENTIAL DIAGNOSIS

ABNORMALITY	DESCRIPTION
Fibrocystic disease	See the table on p. 105.
Fibroadenoma	See the table on p. 105.
Malignant breast tumors	See the table on p. 105.
Adult gynecomastia	Smooth, firm, mobile, tender disk of breast tissue behind areola in males, unilaterally or bilaterally.

SAMPLE DOCUMENTATION

Breasts. Moderate size, conical shaped; left slightly larger than right; granular consistency bilaterally; 1 cm × 2 cm × 3 cm round mass with well-delineated borders at 5 o'clock in left breast, tender, freely mobile in all directions, consistently soft, no dimpling or retraction.

Nipple and areola. Left nipple everted, right inverted (lifetime history); no discharge; areolae dark brown, equal bilaterally with Montgomery tubercles.

Lymph nodes. No supraclavicular or axillary nodes palpable.

Abdomen

EQUIPMENT

♦ Stethoscope
♦ Marking pen
♦ Centimeter ruler or measuring tape
♦ Reflex hammer or tongue blade

EXAMINATION

Have patient in the supine position to start the examination.

TECHNIQUE	FINDINGS
Inspect abdomen in all four quadrants (see the box on p. 108)	
♦ Skin color/characteristics	Expected: Usual color variations, such as paleness or tanning lines. Fine venous network (venous return toward head above umbilicus, toward feet below umbilicus). *Unexpected: Generalized color changes, such as jaundice or cyanosis. Glistening taut appearance. Bluish periumbilical discoloration, bruises, and other localized discoloration. Striae, lesions or nodules, a pearl-like enlarged umbilical node, and scars.*

ANATOMIC CORRELATES OF THE FOUR QUADRANTS OF THE ABDOMEN

Right upper quadrant

Liver and gallbladder
Pylorus
Duodenum
Head of pancreas
Right adrenal gland
Portion of right kidney
Hepatic flexure of colon
Portions of ascending and
    transverse colon

Left upper quadrant

Left lobe of liver
Spleen
Stomach
Body of pancreas
Left adrenal gland
Portion of left kidney
Splenic flexure of colon
Portions of transverse and
    descending colon

Right lower quadrant

Lower pole of right kidney
Cecum and appendix
Portion of ascending colon
Bladder (if distended)
Ovary and salpinx
Uterus (if enlarged)
Right spermatic cord
Right ureter

Left lower quadrant

Lower pole of left kidney
Sigmoid colon
Portion of descending colon
Bladder (if distended)
Ovary and salpinx
Uterus (if enlarged)
Left spermatic cord
Left ureter

TECHNIQUE	FINDINGS
♦ Contour/symmetry Begin seated to patient's right to enhance shadows and contouring. Inspect while patient breathes comfortably and while patient holds a deep breath. Assess symmetry, first seated at patient's side, then standing behind patient's head.	Expected: Flat, rounded, or scaphoid. Contralateral areas symmetric. Maximum height of convexity at umbilicus. Abdomen remains smooth and symmetric while holding breath. In children, the abdomen will be protuberant until age 3. Unexpected: Umbilicus displaced upward, downward, or laterally, or inflamed, swollen, or bulging. Any distention (symmetric or asymmetric), bulges, or masses while breathing comfortably or holding breath.

Technique	Findings
♦ Surface motion	**Expected:** Smooth, even motion with respiration, females mostly costal, males mostly abdominal. Pulsation in upper midline in thin adults. Pulsation in epigastric area in infants. *Unexpected: Limited motion with respiration in adult males. Rippling movement (peristalsis) or marked pulsation.*
Inspect abdominal muscles as patient raises head	**Expected:** No masses or protrusions. *Unexpected: Masses, protrusion of the umbilicus and other hernia signs, or muscle separation.*
Auscultate with stethoscope diaphragm	
♦ Frequency and character of bowel sounds Warm stethoscope diaphragm and hold with light pressure. Auscultate in all quadrants.	**Expected:** 5 to 35 irregular clicks and gurgles per minute. Borborygmi or increased sounds due to hunger. *Unexpected: Increased sounds unrelated to hunger, high-pitched tinkling, or decreased or absent sounds.*
♦ Liver and spleen	**Expected:** Silent. *Unexpected: Friction rubs.*
Auscultate with stethoscope bell	
♦ Vascular sounds Listen with stethoscope bell in all quadrants.	**Expected:** No bruits, venous hum, or friction rubs. *Unexpected: Bruits in aortic, renal, iliac, or femoral arteries.*
♦ Epigastric region and around umbilicus	**Expected:** No venous hum. *Unexpected: Venous hum.*

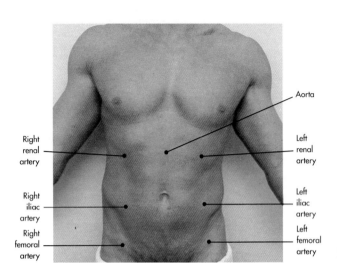

Aorta

Right
renal
artery

Left
renal
artery

Right
iliac
artery

Left
iliac
artery

Right
femoral
artery

Left
femoral
artery

PERCUSSION NOTES OF THE ABDOMEN

Note	Description	Location
Tympany	Musical note of higher pitch than resonance	Over air-filled viscera
Hyperresonance	Pitch lies between tympany and resonance	Base of left lung
Resonance	Sustained note of moderate pitch	Over lung tissue and sometimes over the abdomen
Dullness	Short, high-pitched note with little resonance	Over solid organs adjacent to air-filled structures

Adapted from AH Robins Co.

TECHNIQUE	FINDINGS

Percuss abdomen

NOTE: Percussion can be done independently or concurrently with palpation.

♦ Tone
Pecuss in all quadrants.

Expected: Tympany predominant. Dullness over organs and solid masses. Dullness in suprapubic area from distended bladder. More tympany is present in children than in adults. See the table on p. 110 for percussion notes.
Unexpected: Dullness predominant.

♦ Liver span
Upper edge of liver is detected by percussing at right midclavicular line over area of tympany. To determine lower liver border, percuss upward as shown in the figure at right and mark with pen where tympany changes to dullness. To determine upper liver border, percuss downward as shown and mark change to dullness. Measure the distance between marks to estimate vertical span.

Expected: Lower border usually begins at or slightly below costal margin. Upper border usually begins at fifth to seventh intercostal space. Span generally ranges from 6 to 12 cm.
Unexpected: Lower liver border more than 2 to 3 cm below costal margin. Upper liver border below seventh or above fifth intercostal span. Span greater than 12 cm or less than 6 cm.

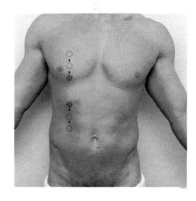

TECHNIQUE	FINDINGS

♦ Spleen
Percuss just posterior to midaxillary line on left, beginning at areas of lung resonance and moving in several directions. Percuss lowest intercostal space in left anterior axillary line before and after patient takes deep breath.

Expected: Small area of dullness from sixth to tenth rib. Tympany before and after deep breath.
Unexpected: Large area of dullness (check for full stomach or feces-filled intestine). Tone change from tympany to dullness with inspiration.

♦ Stomach
Percuss in area of left lower anterior rib cage and left epigastric region.

Expected: Tympany of gastric air bubble (lower than intestine tympany).
Unexpected: Dullness.

Lightly palpate abdomen

Stand at patient's side (usually right). Systematically palpate all quadrants, avoiding areas previously identified as trouble spots. With palmar surfaces of fingers, depress abdominal wall up to 1 cm with light, even motion.
Identify areas of peritoneal irritation by assessing for cutaneous hypersensitivity.

Expected: Abdomen smooth with consistent softness. Possible tension from palpating too deeply, cold hands, or ticklishness.
Unexpected: Muscular tension or resistance, tenderness, or masses. If resistance is present, place pillow under patient's knees, and ask patient to breathe slowly throughout mouth. Feel for relaxation of rectus abdominis muscles on expiration. Continuing tension signals involuntary response to abdominal rigidity. Cutaneous hypersensitivity.

TECHNIQUE	FINDINGS

Palpate abdomen with moderate pressure

Using same hand position as above, palpate all quadrants again, this time with moderate pressure. Using side of hand, palpate liver and spleen through respiratory cycle.

Expected: Liver and spleen palpable during inspiration.
Unexpected: Tenderness.

Deeply palpate abdomen

With same hand position as above, repeat palpation in all quadrants, pressing deeply and evenly into abdominal wall. Move fingers back and forth over abdominal contents. Use bimanual technique—exerting pressure with top hand and concentrating on sensation with bottom hand, as shown in the figure at right—if obesity or muscular resistance makes deep palpation difficult.
To help determine if masses are superficial or intraabdominal, have patient lift head from examining table

Expected: Possible sensation of abdominal wall sliding back and forth. Possible awareness of borders of rectus abdominis muscles, aorta, and portions of colon. Possible tenderness over cecum, sigmoid colon, aorta, and in midline near xiphoid process.
Unexpected: Bulges, masses, and tenderness unrelated to deep palpation of cecum, sigmoid colon, aorta, and xiphoid process. Note location, size, shape, consistency, tenderness, pulsation, mobility, and movement (with respiration) of any masses.

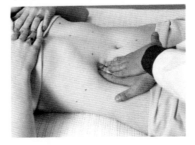

TECHNIQUE	FINDINGS

to contract abdominal muscles and obscure intraabdominal masses.

♦ Umbilical ring and umbilicus
Palpate umbilical ring and around umbilicus. Note whether ring is incomplete or soft in center.

Expected: Umbilical ring circular and free of irregularities. Umbilicus either slightly inverted or everted. Children up to 4 years old may have an umbilical hernia.
Unexpected: Bulges, nodules, and granulation. Protruding umbilicus.

♦ Liver
Place left hand under patient at eleventh and twelfth ribs, lifting to elevate liver toward abdominal wall. Place right hand on abdomen, fingers extended toward head with tips on right midclavicular line below level of liver dullness, as shown in the figure at right. Alternately, place right hand parallel to right costal margin, as shown in the figure at right, below. Press right hand gently but deeply in and up. Ask patient to breathe comfortably a few times and then take a deep breath. Feel for liver edge as diaphragm pushes it down. If palpable, re-

Expected: Usually liver is not palpable. If felt, liver edge should be firm, smooth, and even.
Unexpected: Tenderness, nodules, or irregularity.

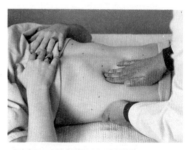

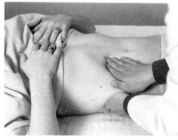

TECHNIQUE

FINDINGS

peat maneuver medi-
ally and laterally to
costal margin. The
liver may be palpable
in young children 2 to
3 cm below the costal
margin. Use light to
moderate pressure.
♦ Gallbladder
Palpate below liver
margin at lateral bor-
der of rectus abdo-
minis muscle.

Expected: Gallbladder not palpable.
Unexpected: *Palpable, tender or*
nontender. If tender (possible
cholecystitis), palpate deeply during
inspiration and observe for pain (Murphy
sign).

♦ Spleen
Reach across patient
with left hand, place it
beneath patient over
left costovertebral an-
gle, and lift spleen an-
teriorly toward ab-
dominal wall. As
shown in the figure,
place right hand on
abdomen below left
costal margin and—
using findings from
percussion—gently
press fingertips inward
toward spleen while
asking patient to take
a deep breath. Feel for
spleen as it moves
downward toward fin-
gers.

Expected: Spleen usually not palpable by either method.
Unexpected: *Palpable spleen.*

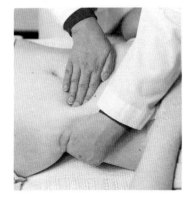

TECHNIQUE   **FINDINGS**

Repeat with patient ly-
ing on right side, as
shown in the figure
below, with hips and
knees flexed. Press in-
ward with left hand
while using fingertips
of right hand to feel
edge of spleen.

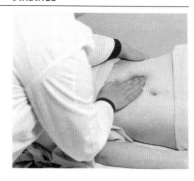

♦ Left kidney
Standing on patient's
right, reach across
with left hand and
place over left flank,
then place right hand
at patient's left costal
margin. Ask patient to
inhale deeply, while
you elevate left flank
and palpate deeply
with right hand.

Expected: Left kidney usually not
palpable.
Unexpected: Pain.

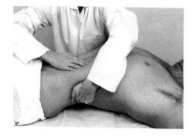

♦ Right kidney
Standing on patient's
right, place left hand
under right flank then
place right hand at pa-
tient's right costal
margin. Ask patient to
inhale deeply while
you elevate right flank
and palpate deeply
with right hand.

Expected: If palpable, right kidney
should be smooth and firm with
rounded edges.
Unexpected: Tenderness.

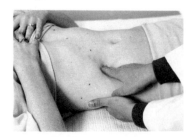

TECHNIQUE	FINDINGS

♦ Aorta
   Palpate deeply slightly to left of midline, and feel for aortic pulsation. As an alternate technique, place palmar surface of hands with fingers extended on midline, as shown in the figure at right, and press fingers deeply inward on each side of aorta and feel for pulsation. For thin patients, use one hand, placing thumb and fingers on either side of aorta.

Expected: Pulsation anterior in direction.
Unexpected: *Prominent lateral pulsation.*

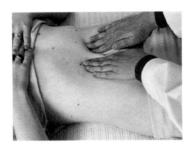

♦ Urinary bladder
   Percuss distended bladder to help determine outline, then palpate.

Expected: Ordinarily not palpable unless distended with urine. If distended, bladder should be smooth, round, and tense, and on percussion will elicit lower note than surrounding air-filled intestines.
Unexpected: *Palpable when not distended with urine.*

Elicit abdominal reflexes

   Stroke each quadrant of abdomen with end of reflex hammer or tongue blade edge. Elicit upper abdominal reflexes by stroking upward and away from umbilicus; elicit lower abdominal reflexes by stroking downward and away from umbilicus.

Expected: With each stroke, contraction of rectus abdominis muscles and pulling of umbilicus toward stroked side. Reflex may be diminished in patient who is obese or whose abdominal muscles were stretched during pregnancy.
Unexpected: *Absence of reflex.*

TECHNIQUE	FINDINGS

With patient sitting, percuss costovertebral angles

Stand behind patient. Right side: Place left hand over right costovertebral angle and strike hand with ulnar surface of left fist. Left side: Repeat with hands reversed.

Expected: No tenderness.
Unexpected: Kidney tenderness or pain.

SOME CAUSES OF PAIN PERCEIVED IN ANATOMIC REGIONS

Right upper quadrant

Duodenal ulcer
Hepatitis
Hepatomegaly
Pneumonia

Left upper quadrant

Ruptured spleen
Gastric ulcer
Aortic aneurysm
Perforated colon
Pneumonia

Right lower quadrant

Appendicitis
Salpingitis
Ovarian cyst
Ruptured ectopic pregnancy
Renal/ureteral stone
Strangulated hernia
Meckel diverticulitis
Regional ileitis
Perforated cecum

Left lower quadrant

Sigmoid diverticulitis
Salpingitis
Ovarian cyst
Ruptured ectopic pregnancy
Renal/ureteral stone
Strangulated hernia
Perforated colon
Regional ileitis
Ulcerative colitis

Periumbilical

Intestinal obstruction
Acute pancreatitis
Early appendicitis
Mesenteric thrombosis
Aortic aneurysm
Diverticulitis

Modified from Judge et al, 1988.

ABNORMALITY	DESCRIPTION

Pain assessment

Keep eyes on patient's face while examining abdomen. To help characterize pain, have patient cough, take a deep breath, jump, or walk. Ask if patient is hungry.

Unexpected: Unwillingness to move, nausea, vomiting, and areas of localized tenderness. Lack of hunger. See the box on p. 118.

Iliopsoas muscle test

Use test for suspected appendicitis. With patient supine, place hand over lower thigh. Ask patient to raise leg, flexing at hip, while you push downward.

Unexpected: Lower quadrant pain.

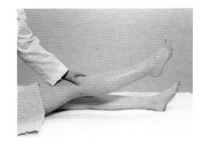

Obturator muscle test

Use test for suspected rupture appendix or pelvic abscess. With patient supine, ask patient to flex right leg at hip and bend knee to 90 degrees. Hold leg just above knee, grasp ankle, and rotate leg laterally and medially, as shown in the figure at right.

Unexpected: Pain in hypogastric region.

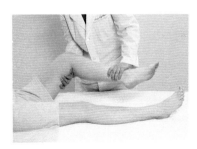

AIDS TO DIFFERENTIAL DIAGNOSIS

ABNORMALITY	DESCRIPTION
Hiatal hernia with esophagitis	Epigastric pain and/or heartburn that worsens with reclining and is relieved by sitting or with antacids; water brash; or dysphagia. Sudden onset of vomiting, pain, and complete dysphagia are symptoms of hernia incarceration.
Duodenal ulcer	Localized epigastric pain occurring with empty stomach that is relieved with food or antacids. Tenderness on palpation of abdomen for anterior-wall ulcers. Hematemesis, melena, dizziness or syncope, decreased blood pressure, increased pulse rate, and decreased hematocrit level are symptoms of upper gastrointestinal bleeding. Signs of an acute abdomen could indicate perforation of duodenum, *a life-threatening event.*
Crohn disease	Cramping diarrhea, mild bleeding, occurs anywhere in GI tract; fissure, fistula abscess formation; periumbilical colic; malabsorption; folate deficiency.
Ulcerative colitis	Mild to severe symptoms; bloody, watery diarrhea; no localized peritoneal signs; weight loss, fatigue, general debility.

ABNORMALITY	DESCRIPTION
Colon cancer	Occult blood in stool. History of changes in frequency or character of stool. Lesion felt on rectal examination. Tumor palpated in right or left lower quadrant.
Hepatitis	Anorexia, vague abdominal pain, nausea, vomiting, malaise, fever, transient skin rashes, and jaundice. Enlarged liver and spleen are classic findings.
Cirrhosis	Ascites, jaundice, prominent abdominal vasculature, cutaneous spider angiomas, dark urine, light-colored stools, and spleen enlargement. Complaints of fatigue. Muscle wasting in late stages.
Cholecystitis	*Acute*: Pain in upper right quadrant with radiation around midtorso to right scapular region. Pain abrupt and severe, lasting 2 to 4 hours. *Chronic*: Repeated acute attacks; a scarred and contracted gallbladder; fat intolerance, flatulence, nausea, anorexia, and nonspecific abdominal pain and tenderness of right hypochondriac region.
Chronic pancreatitis	Unremitting abdominal pain, epigastric tenderness, weight loss, steatorrhea, and glucose intolerance.

ABNORMALITY	DESCRIPTION
Pyelonephritis	Flank pain, bacteriuria, pyuria, dysuria, nocturia, and urinary frequency. Possible costovertebral angle tenderness.
Renal calculi	Fever, hematuria, and flank pain that may extend to groin and genitals.
Appendicitis	Initially, periumbilical or epigastric pain; colicky; later becomes localized to RLQ, often at McBurney point.

SAMPLE DOCUMENTATION

Abdomen rounded and symmetric without distention; no lesions, scars, or visible peristalsis; silver striae over lower quadrants; aorta midline without bruit or visible pulsation; umbilicus inverted and midline without herniation; bowel sounds heard in all quadrants; renal, iliac, and femoral arteries without bruits; tympanic percussion tones over epigastrium, remainder resonant to percussion; soft and relaxed without tenderness or masses; liverspan 8 cm at MCL, 6 cm at MSL, nontender; gallbladder, spleen, and kidneys not palpable; superficial reflexes intact; no CVA tenderness.

Female Genitalia

EQUIPMENT

♦ Gloves
♦ Sterile cotton swabs
♦ Culture plates
♦ Cytologic fixative
♦ Speculum
♦ Water-soluble lubricant

♦ Lamp
♦ Wooden or plastic spatula
♦ Glass slides
♦ Cervical brushes
♦ Chlamydial enzyme immunoassay kit

EXAMINATION

Have patient in lithotomy position, draped for minimal exposure.

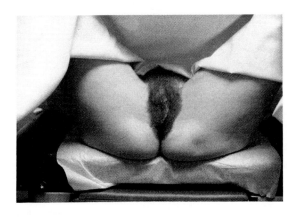

TECHNIQUE	FINDINGS

External Genitalia
Wear gloves on both hands.

Ask patient to separate or spread legs. Tell patient you are beginning examination, then touch either lower thigh and—without breaking contact—move hand along thigh to external genitalia.

Examine the infant using the frog leg position.

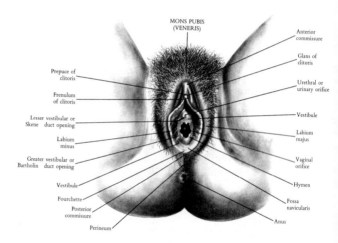

MONS PUBIS (VENERIS)

Prepuce of clitoris

Frenulum of clitoris

Lesser vestibular or Skene duct opening

Labium minus

Greater vestibular or Bartholin duct opening

Vestibule

Fourchette

Posterior commissure

Perineum

Anterior commissure

Glans of clitoris

Urethral or urinary orifice

Vestibule

Labium majus

Vaginal orifice

Hymen

Fossa navicularis

Anus

Inspect and palpate mons pubis

♦ Characteristics

Expected: Skin smooth and clean.
Unexpected: Improper hygiene.

♦ Pubic hair

Expected: Regularly distributed female pubic hair.
Unexpected: Nits or lice.

TECHNIQUE	FINDINGS
Inspect and palpate labia	
♦ Labia majora	**Expected:** Gaping or closed, dry or moist, shriveled or full, tissue soft and homogeneous, usually symmetric. **Unexpected:** *Swelling, redness, tenderness, discoloration, varicosities, obvious stretching, or signs of trauma or scarring. If excoriation, rashes, or lesions are present, ask patient if she has been scratching.*
♦ Labia minora Separate labia majora with fingers of one hand. With other hand, palpate labia minora between thumb and second finger.	**Expected:** Symmetric with moist, dark-pink inner surface. Tissue soft and homogeneous. **Unexpected:** *Tenderness, inflammation, irritation, excoriation, caking of discharge in tissue folds, discoloration, ulcers, vesicles, irregularities, or nodules. Hyperemia of fourchette not related to recent sexual activity.*
Inspect clitoris	
♦ Size and length	**Expected:** Length 2 cm or less; diameter 0.5 cm. The clitoris of a term infant is usually covered by labia minora and may appear relatively large. **Unexpected:** *Enlargement, atrophy, inflammation, or adhesions.*
Inspect urethral meatus and vaginal opening	
♦ Urethral orifice	**Expected:** Slit or irregular opening, close to or in vaginal introitus, and usually midline. **Unexpected:** *Discharge, polyps, caruncles, fistulas, lesions, irritation, inflammation, or dilation.*

TECHNIQUE	FINDINGS
♦ Vaginal introitus	**Expected:** Thin vertical slit or large orifice with irregular edges. Tissue moist. *Unexpected: Swelling, discoloration, discharge, lesions, fistulas, or fissures.*
♦ Inspect for discharge in infants and children	**Expected:** Mucoid whitish vaginal discharge may be mixed with blood until 4 weeks of age. *Unexpected: Mucoid discharge from irritation by diapers or powder; any discharge in children.*

Milk Skene glands

Tell patient you will be inserting one finger in her vagina and pressing forward with it. With palm up, insert index finger to second joint, press upward, and milk Skene glands by moving finger outward. Perform on both sides of urethra and directly on urethra.

Unexpected: Discharge or tenderness. Note color, consistency, and odor of any discharge; obtain culture.

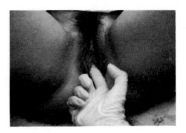

Palpate Bartholin glands

Tell patient she will feel you pressing around entrance to vagina. Palpate lateral tissue between index finger and thumb, then palpate entire area bilaterally, particularly posterolateral portion of labia majora.

Expected: No swelling.
Unexpected: Swelling, tenderness, masses, heat, fluctuation, or discharge. Note color, consistency, and odor of any discharge; obtain culture.

TECHNIQUE	FINDINGS

Test vaginal muscle tone

Ask patient to squeeze vaginal opening around your finger.

Expected: Fairly tight squeezing by some nulliparous women, less so by some multiparous women.
Unexpected: Protrusion of cervix or uterus.

Inspect for bulging and urinary incontinence

Ask patient to bear down.

Expected: No bulging.
Unexpected: Bulging of anterior of posterior wall, or urinary incontinence.

Inspect and palpate perineum

Compress perineum tissue between finger and thumb.

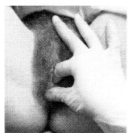

Expected: Perineum surface smooth—generally thick and smooth in a nulliparous woman, thinner and rigid in a multiparous woman. Possible episiotomy scarring in women who have borne children.
Unexpected: Tenderness, inflammation, fistulas, lesions, or growths.

Inspect anus

♦ Skin characteristics

Expected: Skin darkly pigmented and possibly coarse.
Unexpected: Scarring, lesions, inflammation, fissures, lumps, skin tags, or excoriation.

Internal Genitalia—Speculum Examination

If you touched the perineum or anal skin while examining the external genitalia, change gloves before beginning internal examination.

Lubricate speculum and gloved fingers with water (if you expect to take specimens for analysis) or water-soluble lubricant (if you do not).

Insert speculum

Tell patient she will feel you touching her again, then insert two fingers of the hand not holding the speculum just inside vaginal introitus and press downward. Ask the patient to breathe slowly and try to consciously relax her muscles. When you feel the muscles relax, insert closed speculum obliquely rotated over your two fingers, directed 45-degrees downward.

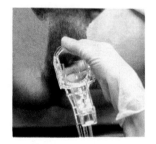

Remove fingers and rotate speculum until it is horizontal, and insert it the length of the vaginal canal. Maintaining downward pressure, open speculum by pressing on thumb piece. Sweep speculum slowly upward until cervix comes into view. Adjust light, then manipulate speculum farther into

TECHNIQUE	FINDINGS

vagina so that cervix is well exposed between anterior and posterior blades. Stabilize distal spread of blades and adjust proximal spread as needed.

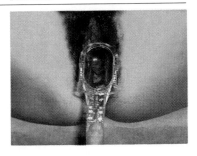

Inspect cervix

♦ Color

Expected: Evenly distributed pink. Symmetric, circumscribed erythema around os can be expected.
Unexpected: *Bluish, pale, or reddened cervix (especially if patchy or with irregular borders).*

♦ Position

Expected: In midline, horizontal or pointing anteriorly or posteriorly. Protruding into vagina 1 to 3 cm.
Unexpected: *Deviation to right or left. Protrusion into vagina greater than 1 to 3 cm.*

♦ Size

Expected: 3 cm in diameter.
Unexpected: *Larger than 3 cm.*

♦ Shape

Expected: Uniform.
Unexpected: *Distorted.*

♦ Surface characteristics

Expected: Surface smooth. Possible symmetric, reddened circle around os (squamocolumnar epithelium). Possible small, white, or yellow, raised round areas on cervix (nabothian cysts).
Unexpected: *Friable tissue, red patchy areas, granular areas, or white patches.*

TECHNIQUE	FINDINGS

♦ Discharge
  Note any discharge.
  Determine origin:
  cervix or vagina.

Expected: Odorless, creamy or clear, thick, thin, or stringy (often heavier at midcycle or immediately before menstruation).
Unexpected: Odorous and white to yellow, green, or gray.

♦ Size and shape of os

Expected: Nulliparous woman: small, round, oval.
Multiparous woman: usually a horizontal slit or irregular and stellate.
Unexpected: Slit resulting from trauma from induced abortion, difficult removal of intrauterine device (IUD), or sexual abuse.

Collect vaginal smears and cultures

Follow CDC guidelines for safe collection of human secretions.

♦ Pap smear
  As shown in the figure at right, collect sample from ectocervix with spatula. Insert longer projection of spatula into cervical os, rotate 360 degrees while keeping it flush against cervical tissue, then withdraw. Spread specimen on glass slide, spray with cytologic fixative, and label.
  Insert brush device into cervical os until only bristles closest to

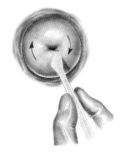

TECHNIQUE	FINDINGS

handle are exposed, rotate ½ to 1 turn, then withdraw. Roll and twist brush across glass slide, spray with cytologic fixative, and label. Warn patient that blood spotting might occur. (Vary technique appropriately for different types of brushes.)

♦ Gonococcal culture specimen
Insert sterile cotton swab into cervical os, hold in place for 10 to 30 seconds, then withdraw. Rotating swab, spread specimen in large **Z** pattern over culture medium and label. Follow agency routine for warming and transporting specimen.
If indicated, obtain anal culture: Insert fresh sterile cotton swab about 2.5 cm into rectum, rotate 360 degrees, hold for 10 to 30 seconds, and withdraw. Rotating swab, spread specimen in large **Z** pattern over culture medium and label.

TECHNIQUE	FINDINGS

♦ Chlamydial enzyme immunoassay specimen
Remove excess mucus from ectocervix with swab and discard. Insert swab specified or provided by kit into cervical os and rotate for 15 to 30 seconds, then withdraw (avoiding vaginal walls). Place in transport tube, with swab in contact with reagent, and label. Follow agency procedure for testing, storage, and shipping.

Withdraw speculum and inspect vaginal walls

Unlock speculum and remove it slowly, rotating it so vaginal walls can be inspected.
Maintain downward pressure and hook index finger over anterior blade as it is removed. Note odor of any discharge pooled in posterior blade, and obtain specimen if not already obtained.

Expected: Vaginal wall color same pink as cervix or lighter; moist, smooth or rugated; and homogeneous. Thin, clear or cloudy; odorless secretions.
Unexpected: Reddened patches, lesions, pallor, cracks, bleeding, nodules, and swelling. Secretions that are profuse; thick, curdy, or frothy; gray, green, or yellow; or malodorous.

| TECHNIQUE | FINDINGS |

Internal Genitalia—Bimanual Examination

Change gloves, and then lubricate index and middle fingers of examining hand.

Tell patient you are going to examine her internally with your fingers. *Prevent thumb from touching clitoris during examination.*

Palpate vaginal wall while inserting fingers into vagina.

Insert tips of index and middle fingers into vaginal opening and press downward, waiting for muscles to relax. Gradually insert fingers full length while palpating vaginal wall.

Expected: Smooth and homogeneous.
Unexpected: Tenderness, lesions, cysts, nodules, masses, or growths.

Palpate cervix

Locate cervix with palmar surface of fingers, feel end, and run fingers around circumference to feel fornices.

♦ Size, shape and length

Expected: Consistent with speculum examination.

♦ Consistency

Expected: Firm in nonpregnant woman; softer in pregnant woman.
Unexpected: Nodules, hardness, or roughness.

♦ Position

Expected: In midline horizontal or pointing anteriorly or posteriorly. Protruding into vagina 1 to 3 cm.
Unexpected: Deviation to right or left. Protrusion into vagina greater than 1 to 3 cm.

TECHNIQUE	FINDINGS
♦ Mobility Grasp cervix gently between fingers and move from side to side. Observe patient's facial expression.	**Expected:** 1 to 2 cm movement in each direction. *Unexpected: Pain or discomfort on movement.*
♦ Patency of cervical os Gently insert fingertip into os.	**Expected:** Fingertip enters os 0.5 cm.

Palpate uterus

♦ Location and position
Place palmar surface of outside hand on abdominal midline, halfway between umbilicus and symphysis pubis, and place intravaginal fingers in anterior fornix. As shown in the figure at right, slowly slide outside hand toward pubis while pressing down and forward with flat surface of fingers; at the same time, push inward and up with fingertips of intravaginal hand while pushing down on cervix with backs of fingers. If uterus is anteverted or anteflexed, you should feel fundus between fingers of two hands at level of pubis.

Expected: In midline, horizontal or pointing anteriorly or posteriorly. Protruding into vagina 1 to 3 cm.
Unexpected: Deviation to right or left. Protrusion into vagina greater than 1 to 3 cm.

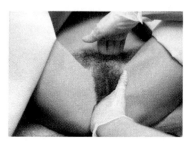

TECHNIQUE   **FINDINGS**

If uterus cannot be felt
with this maneuver,
place intravaginal fin-
gers together in poste-
rior fornix and outside
hand immediately
above symphysis pu-
bis. Press firmly down
with outside hand
while pressing inward
against cervix with in-
travaginal hand. If
uterus is retroverted
or retroflexed, you
should feel fundus.
If uterus cannot be felt
with either of these
maneuvers, move in-
travaginal fingers to
each side of cervix
and, while keeping
contact with cervix,
press inward and feel
as far as possible.
Slide fingers so they
are on top and bottom
of cervix and continue
pressing in while mov-
ing fingers to feel as
much of uterus as
possible. (When
uterus is in midposi-
tion, you will not be
able to feel it with out-
side hand.)

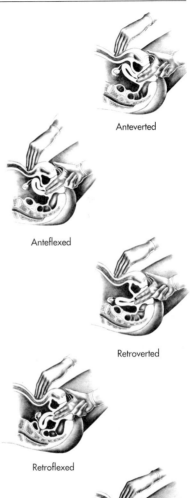

Anteverted

Anteflexed

Retroverted

Retroflexed

Midposition

TECHNIQUE	FINDINGS
◆ Size, shape, and contour	**Expected:** Pear shaped and 5.5 to 8.0 cm long (larger in all dimensions in multiparous women). Contour rounded and, in nonpregnant women, walls firm and smooth. *Unexpected: Larger than expected or interrupted contour or smoothness.*
◆ Mobility Gently move uterus between intravaginal fingers and outside hand.	**Expected:** Mobile in anteroposterior plane. *Unexpected: Fixed uterus or tenderness on movement.*

Palpate ovaries

Place fingers of outside hand on lower right quadrant. With intravaginal hand facing up, place both fingers in right lateral fornix. Press intravaginal fingers deeply in and up toward abdominal hand, while sweeping flat surface of fingers of outside hand deeply in and obliquely down toward symphysis pubis. Palpate entire area by firmly pressing outside hand and intravaginal fingers together.
Repeat on left side.

◆ Consistency

Expected: If palpable, ovaries should feel firm, smooth, and slightly to moderately tender. *Unexpected: Marked tenderness or nodularity. Palpable fallopian tubes.*

TECHNIQUE	FINDINGS
♦ Size	**Expected:** About 3 cm × 2 cm × 1 cm.
	Unexpected: Enlargement.
♦ Shape	**Expected:** Ovoid.

Palpate adnexal areas

Use hand positions for palpating ovaries.

Expected: Adnexae difficult to palpate.
Unexpected: Masses and tenderness. If adnexal masses are found, characterize by size, shape, location, consistency, and tenderness.

Internal Genitalia—Rectovaginal Examination

Change gloves.

This examination may be uncomfortable for the patient. Assure her that although she may feel the urgency of a bowel movement, she will not have one. Ask her to breathe slowly and try to relax her sphincter, rectum, and buttocks.

Insert index finger into vagina and middle finger into anus

To insert middle finger into anus, press against anus and ask patient to bear down. As she does, slip tip of finger into rectum just past sphincter.

Assess sphincter tone

Palpate area or anorectal junction and just above it. Ask patient to tighten and relax anal sphincter.

Expected: Even sphincter tightening.
Unexpected: Extremely tight, lax, or absent sphincter.

TECHNIQUE	FINDINGS

Palpate anterior rectal wall and rectovaginal septum

Slide both fingers in as far as possible, then ask patient to bear down. Rotate rectal finger to explore anterior rectal wall and palpate rectovaginal septum.

Expected: Smooth and uninterrupted. Uterine body and uterine fundus sometimes felt with retroflexed uterus.
Unexpected: *Masses, polyps, nodules, strictures, and irregularities, and tenderness.*

Palpate posterior aspect of uterus

Place outside hand just above symphysis pubis and press firmly and deeply down, while positioning intravaginal finger in posterior vaginal fornix and pressing strongly upward against posterior side of cervix, as shown in the figure at right. Palpate as much of posterior side of uterus as possible.

Expected: Consistent with bimanual examination regarding location, position, size, shape, and contour.
Unexpected: *Tenderness.*

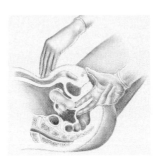

Palpate posterior rectal wall

As you withdraw fingers, rotate intrarectal finger to evaluate posterior rectal wall.

Expected: Smooth and uninterrupted.
Unexpected: *Masses, polyps, nodules, strictures, irregularities, and tenderness.*

ABNORMALITY	FINDINGS
Note characteristics of feces when gloved finger removed	**Expected:** Light to dark brown in color. *Unexpected:* Blood. *Note color of any blood and prepare specimen for guiac testing.*
Wipe patient's perineum, using front-to-back stroke and clean tissue for each stroke	

AIDS TO DIFFERENTIAL DIAGNOSIS

ABNORMALITY	DESCRIPTION
Premenstrual syndrome (PMS)	Edema, headache, weight gain, and behavior disturbances such as irritability, nervousness, dysphoria, and lack of coordination. Symptoms occur 5 to 7 days before menses, then subside.
Endometriosis	Pelvic pain, dysmenorrhea, and heavy or prolonged menstrual flow.
Condyloma acuminatum (genital warts)	Warty lesions on labia, within vestibule, or in perianal region. The growths (generally whitish-pink to reddish-brown, discrete, and soft) may occur singly or in clusters, and may enlarge to cauliflower masses.
Herpes lesions	Small, red vesicles that may itch and usually are painful. Initial infection often extensive; recurrent infection normally a localized patch on vulva, perineum, vagina, or cervix.

VAGINAL INFECTIONS

Microorganisms	Discharge	Erythema/itching	Associated symptoms	Diagnosis
Neisseria gonorrhoeae	Yellow/green or may be absent; from cervical os	Cervix and vulva may be inflamed	Dysuria, frequency; discharge from Skene glands on milking; symptoms of PID may be present	Culture
Chlamydia trachomatis	Most infections are asymptomatic; may have yellow mucopurulent discharge from cervical os; occurs with gonococcal infection, urethritis, mucopurulent cervicitis, and PID	Hypertrophic, edematous, friable area of cervical ectopy	Intermenstrual spotting, spotting after intercourse, asymptomatic urethritis, Bartholin gland discharge	Tissue culture; chlamydia enzyme immunoassay; fluorescein-labeled monoclonal antibody tests

VAGINAL INFECTIONS—Cont'd

Microorganisms	Discharge	Erythema/itching	Associated symptoms	Diagnosis
Candida albicans	Scant to moderate; may be thin but usually thick, white, curdy, adherent	Mild to severe itching and erythema of labia, thighs, perineum; cervix may be red and edematous	Dysuria, frequency, dyspareunia	Potassium hydroxide (KOH) shows mycelia, spores
Trichomonas vaginalis	Copious, frothy, gray/green; strong, foul odor	Severe itching of vulva, with or without erythema; petechiae of cervix and vagina ("strawberry spots")	Dysuria and dyspareunia with severe infection	Wet mount shows large number of polymorphonuclear neutrophils (PMNs) and trichomonads
Gardnerella (*Haemophilus*) *vaginalis*	Scant or moderate; homogeneous, grey, foul odor	Mild or absent	Strong fishy vaginal odor, particularly after intercourse	Wet mount shows "clue cells"

ABNORMALITY	DESCRIPTION
Vaginal infections	Often vaginal discharge, possibly accompanied by urinary symptoms. Sometimes asymptomatic (see the table on p. 140).
Cervical carcinoma	Hard granular surface at or near cervical os. Lesion can evolve to form extensive, irregular, easily bleeding cauliflower growth.
Uterine bleeding	See the table below.
Pelvic inflammatory disease (PID)	Acute PID: very tender bilateral adnexal areas. Chronic PID: bilateral tender, irregular, and fairly fixed adnexal areas.

TYPES OF UTERINE BLEEDING AND ASSOCIATED CAUSES

Type	Common causes
Midcycle spotting	Midcycle estradiol fluctuation associated with ovulation
Delayed menstruation with excessive bleeding	Anovulation or threatened abortion
Frequent bleeding	Chronic PID, endometriosis, DUB,* anovulation
Profuse menstrual bleeding	Endometrial polyps, DUB, adenomyosis, submucous leiomyomas, IUD
Intermenstrual or irregular bleeding	Endometrial polyps, DUB, uterine or cervical cancer, oral contraceptives
Postmenopausal bleeding	Endometrial hyperplasia, estrogen therapy, endometrial cancer

*Modified from Thompson et al, 1993.
*DUB, Dysfunctional uterine bleeding.

SAMPLE DOCUMENTATION

External. Female hair distribution; no masses, lesions, scars, rashes, or swelling of vulva; labia, clitoris, vaginal orifice, and urethral meatus intact without discharge, inflammation, or tenderness; perineum intact and nontender, healed episiotomy scar present.

Internal—Speculum. Vaginal mucosa moist and pink without lesions, odor, or discharge; cervix pink, smooth, midline, points posteriorly, no lesions; os horizontal slit.

Internal—Bimanual. Vaginal walls smooth, nontender; cervix smooth, firm, mobile, nontender; os patent; uterus midline, anteverted, firm, smooth, approximately 9 cm long, nontender; right ovary palpable, approximately 3 cm × 2 cm × 1 cm, slightly tender; left ovary not palpable, nontender; no adnexal masses.

Internal—Rectovaginal. Sacrococcygeal and perianal area intact without lesions, rashes, inflammation, excoriation, or scars; anal hemorrhoids; sphincter tightens evenly; anal ring smooth and intact; rectal walls smooth and even without nodules, polyps, tenderness; rectovaginal septum intact; guaiac negative.

....

12

Male Genitalia

EQUIPMENT

♦ Gloves

EXAMINATION

Have patient lying or standing to start the examination.
Wear gloves.

TECHNIQUE	FINDINGS
Inspect pubic hair	
♦ Characteristics	Expected: Coarser than scalp hair.
♦ Distribution	Expected: Male hair distribution. Abundant in pubic region, continuing around scrotum to anal orifice, and possibly continuing in narrowing midline to umbilicus. Penis without hair; scrotum with scant hair.

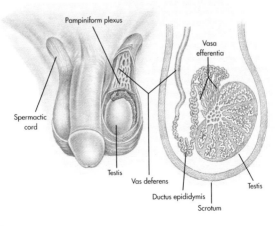

Pampiniform plexus

Vasa efferentia

Spermactic cord

Testis

Vas deferens

Ductus epididymis

Scrotum

Testis

TECHNIQUE	FINDINGS
Inspect glans penis	
♦ Uncircumcised patient Retract foreskin	**Expected:** Dorsal vein apparent. Foreskin easily retracted. In children the foreskin is fully retractable by age 3 to 4 years. White, cheesy smegma visible over glans. *Unexpected: Tight foreskin (phimosis). Lesions or discharge.*
♦ Circumcised patient	**Expected:** Dorsal vein apparent. Exposed glans erythematous and dry. *Unexpected: Lesions or discharge.*
Examine external meatus of urethra (foreskin retracted in uncircumcised patient)	
♦ Shape	**Expected:** Slitlike opening. *Unexpected: Pinpoint or round opening.*
♦ Location	**Expected:** On ventral surface and only millimeters from tip of glans. *Unexpected: Any place other than tip of glans or along shaft of penis.*
♦ Urethral orifice Press glans between thumb and forefinger.	**Expected:** Opening glistening and pink. *Unexpected: Bright erythema or discharge.*
Palpate penis	**Expected:** Soft (flaccid penis). *Unexpected: Tenderness, induration, or nodularity. Prolonged erection (priapism).*
Strip urethra Firmly compress base of penis with thumb and forefinger; move toward glans.	*Unexpected: Discharge.*

TECHNIQUE	FINDINGS

Inspect scrotum and ventral surface of penis

♦ Color

Expected: Darker than body skin and often reddened in red-haired patients.
Unexpected: Reddened in patients without red hair.

♦ Texture

Expected: Surface possibly coarse. Small lumps on scrotal skin (sebaceous or epidermoid cysts) that sometimes discharge oily material.

♦ Shape

Expected: Asymmetry. Thickness varying with temperature, age, and emotional state.
Unexpected: Unusual thickening, often with pitting.

Palpate inguinal canal for direct or indirect hernia

With patient standing, ask him to bear down as if for bowel movement. While he strains, inspect area of inguinal canal and region of fossa ovalis. Ask patient to relax, and insert examining finger into lower part of scrotum and carry upward along vas deferens into inguinal canal, as shown in the figure at right. Ask patient to cough. Repeat examination on opposite side.

Expected: Presence of oval external ring.
Unexpected: Feeling a viscus against examining finger with coughing. If hernia felt, note as indirect (felt within inguinal canal or even into scrotum) or direct (felt medial to external canal).

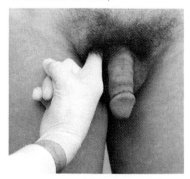

TECHNIQUE	FINDINGS

Palpate testes

Use thumb and first
two fingers.

♦ Consistency

Expected: Smooth and rubbery.
Sensitive to gentle compression.
Unexpected: Tenderness or nodules.
Total insensitivity to painful stimuli.

♦ Texture

Unexpected: Irregular texture.

♦ Size

Unexpected: Irregular size; asymmetry
in size, <1 cm or >5 cm.

♦ Descension
Palpate testes in chil-
dren to determine if
testes have de-
scended.

Expected: Bilaterally palpable; 1
cm in size. Considered descended if
testis can be pushed into scrotum.

Palpate epididymides

Expected: Smooth and discrete,
with the larger part cephalad.
Unexpected: Tenderness.

Palpate vasa deferentia

Palpate from testicle
to inguinal ring. Re-
peat with other testi-
cle.

Expected: Smooth and discrete.
Unexpected: Beaded or lumpy.

Palpate for inguinal lymph nodes

Ask patient to lie
supine, with knee
slightly flexed on side
of palpation.

Expected: Nodes accessible to palpation, but not large enough or
firm enough to be felt.
Unexpected: Enlarged, tender, red or
discolored, fixed, matted, inflamed, or
warm nodes and increased
vascularity.

Elicit cremasteric reflex bilaterally

Stroke inner thigh with
blunt instrument. Re-
peat with other thigh.

Expected: Testicle and scrotum on
stroked side rise.

AIDS TO DIFFERENTIAL DIAGNOSIS

ABNORMALITY	DESCRIPTION
Herpes	Superficial vesicles—located on glans, penile shaft, or base of penis—that are frequently quite painful. Often associated with inguinal lymphadenopathy and systemic symptoms (e.g., fever) in primary infection.
Hernia	See the table on p. 149.
Hydrocele	Nontender, smooth, firm mass in scrotum.
Varicocele	Abnormal tortuosity and dilated veins of pampiniform plexus within spermatic cord. Generally on left side and sometimes painful.
Epididymitis	Pain and possible erythema of overlying scrotum. ***Fever and white blood cells and bacteria in urine suggest testicular torsion, a surgical emergency.*** In chronic form, epididymis feels firm and lumpy and may be slightly tender, and vasa deferentia may be beaded.
Priapism	Prolonged painful penile erection. Can occur in patients with leukemia or sickle cell disease.
Hypospadias	Urethral meatus is located on ventral surface of glans, penile shaft, or perineal area.
Epispadias	Urethral meatus is located on dorsal surface of the penile shaft.

DISTINGUISHING CHARACTERISTICS OF HERNIAS

	Indirect inguinal	Direct inguinal	Femoral
Incidence	Most common type of hernia; both sexes are affected; often patients are children and young males	Less common than indirect inguinal; occurs more often in males than females; more common in those after age 40	Least common type of hernia; occurs more often in females than males; rare in children
Occurrence	Through internal inguinal ring; can remain in canal, exit the external ring, or pass into scrotum; may be bilateral	Through external inguinal ring; located in region of Hesselbach triangle; rarely enters scrotum	Through femoral ring, femoral canal, and fossa ovalis
Presentation	Soft swelling in area of internal ring; pain on straining; hernia comes down canal and touches fingertip on examination	Bulge in area of Hesselbach triangle; usually painless; easily reduced; hernia bulges anteriorly, pushes against side of finger on examination	Right side presentation more common than left; pain may be severe; inguinal canal empty on examination

SAMPLE DOCUMENTATION

Pubic hair in male pattern. Circumcised penis smooth, with no lesions, induration, or discharge. Meatal slit patent, on ventral surface at tip of glans. Scrotal contents smooth without tenderness, swelling, or masses. Inguinal areas smooth, no lymph nodes palpable. Inguinal canals without masses, bulges, or tenderness. Cremasteric reflex present.

13

Anus, Rectum, and Prostate

EQUIPMENT

♦ Gloves
♦ Water-soluble lubricant
♦ Penlight
♦ Sterile cotton swabs
♦ Culture plates
♦ Cytologic fixative

EXAMINATION

Have patient in knee-chest, left lateral position with hips and knees flexed, or standing with hips flexed and upper body supported by examining table.

Wear gloves on one or both hands.

TECHNIQUE	FINDINGS
Inspect and palpate sacrococcygeal and perianal area	
♦ Skin characteristics	**Expected:** Smooth and uninterrupted. **Unexpected:** *Lumps, rashes, tenderness, inflammation, excoriation, pilonidal dimpling, or tufts of hair.*
Inspect anus	
♦ Spread patient's buttocks. Examine, using penlight or lamp if needed, with patient relaxed as well as with patient bearing down.	

TECHNIQUE	FINDINGS

♦ Skin characteristics

Expected: Skin coarser and darker than on buttocks.

Unexpected: Skin lesions, skin tags or warts, external or internal hemorrhoids, fissures, and fistulas, rectal prolapse, or polyps. Describe any irregularities and locate using clock referents (12 o'clock ventral midline/6 o'clock dorsal midline).

Insert finger and assess sphincter tone

Put water-soluble lubricant on index finger; press pad against anal opening and ask patient to bear down to relax external sphincter. As relaxation occurs, slip tip of finger into anal canal, as shown in the figure at right. (Assure patient that although he or she may feel the urgency of a bowel movement, it will not occur.) Ask patient to tighten external sphincter around finger.

Expected: Even sphincter tightening.

Unexpected: Patient discomfort. Lax or extremely tight sphincter, tenderness.

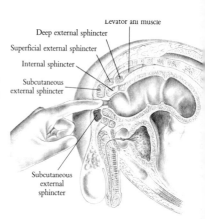

Levator ani muscle
Deep external sphincter
Superficial external sphincter
Internal sphincter
Subcutaneous external sphincter
Subcutaneous external sphincter

Palpate muscular anal ring

Rotate finger.

Expected: Smooth and even with consistent pressure exerted.

Unexpected: Nodules or other irregularities.

TECHNIQUE	FINDINGS

Palpate lateral and posterior rectal walls

Insert finger farther and rotate to palpate the lateral, then posterior, rectal walls. (If helpful, perform bidigital palpation with thumb and index finger by lightly pressing thumb against perianal tissue and bringing index finger toward thumb.)

Expected: Smooth, even, and uninterrupted.
Unexpected: Nodules, masses, polyps, tenderness, or irregularities. (Internal hemorrhoids not ordinarily felt unless thrombosed.)

Males: Palpate posterior surface of prostate gland through anterior rectal wall

Rotate finger and palpate anterior rectal wall and the posterior surface of prostate gland. (Alert patient that he may feel urge to urinate but won't.)

♦ Consistency and characteristics of anterior rectal wall

Expected: Smooth, even, and uninterrupted.
Unexpected: Nodules, masses, polyps, tenderness, or irregularities.

♦ Consistency, contour, and characteristics of prostate

Expected: Surface firm and smooth, lateral lobes symmetric, median sulcus palpable, and seminal vesicles not palpable.
Unexpected: Rubberiness, bogginess, fluctuant softness, stony hard nodularity, tenderness, obliterated sulcus, or palpable seminal vesicles.

TECHNIQUE	FINDINGS
♦ Mobility of prostate gland	**Expected:** Slightly movable.
♦ Size of prostate gland	**Expected:** 4 cm diameter with less than 1 cm protruding into rectum. *Unexpected: Protrusion greater than 1 cm (note distance of protrusion).* *Unexpected: Discharge that appears at urethral meatus (collect specimen for microscopic examination).*
Females: Palpate cervix and uterus through anterior rectal wall	
Attempt to palpate cervix through anterior rectal wall.	
♦ Size	**Expected:** 3 cm in diameter. *Unexpected: Larger than 3 cm in diameter.*
♦ Shape	*Unexpected: Distorted.*
♦ Position	**Expected:** In midline, horizontal or pointing anteriorly or posteriorly. *Unexpected: Deviation to right or left.*
♦ Surface characteristics	**Expected:** Smooth. *Unexpected: Friable or irregular.*
♦ Mobility	**Expected:** 1 to 2 cm movement in each direction. *Unexpected: Pain or discomfort on movement.*
Have patient bear down, and palpate deeper	
Ask patient to bear down while you reach farther into rectum. Females: explore in cul-de-sac. Males: explore above prostate.	*Unexpected: Tenderness of peritoneal area or nodules.*

TECHNIQUE	FINDINGS
Withdraw finger and examine fecal material	
♦ Color and consistency	**Expected:** Soft and brown. **Unexpected:** *Blood, pus, or light-tan, gray, or tarry-black stool. Test any fecal material for blood using chemical guaiac procedure.*

AIDS TO DIFFERENTIAL DIAGNOSIS

ABNORMALITY	DESCRIPTION
Perianal and perirectal abscesses	Pain and tenderness in anal area, usually accompanied by a fever.
Enterobiasis infestation in children	Intense perianal itching, especially at night.
Anorectal fissure and fistula	Fissure: Pain, itching, or bleeding, with spastic internal sphincter. Fistula: Elevated, red, granular tissue at external opening, possibly with serosanguinous or purulent drainage on compression of the area.
Hemorrhoids	External: Itching and bleeding with defecation. Thrombosed hemorrhoids appear as blue, shiny masses at anus. Internal: Bleeding with or without defecation. Do not cause discomfort unless thrombosed, prolapsed, or infected.
Rectal carcinoma	Generally asymptomatic.
Prostatic carcinoma	On rectal examination, a hard irregular nodule may be palpable. Prostate feels asymmetric and median sulcus is obliterated in advanced carcinoma.

ABNORMALITY	DESCRIPTION
Benign prostatic hypertrophy	Hesitancy on urination, decreased force and caliber of stream, dribbling, incomplete emptying of bladder, nocturia, and dysuria.

SAMPLE DOCUMENTATION

Anus/rectum. Sacrococcygeal and perianal area intact without lesions, rashes, inflammation, excoriation, or scars; anal surface intact without lesions, fissures, or fistulas; external hemorrhoid at 4 o'clock position, painful, not bleeding; sphincter tightens evenly; anal ring smooth and intact; rectal walls smooth and even, without nodules, polyps, tenderness; guaiac negative.

Prostate. Lateral lobes symmetric, smooth, rubbery; sulcus not palpable; grade II protrusion; nontender.

CHAPTER

14

Musculoskeletal System

EQUIPMENT

- ♦ Goniometer
- ♦ Skin-marking pencil
- ♦ Reflex hammer
- ♦ Tape measure

EXAMINATION

Begin examination as patient enters room, observing gait and posture. During examination, note how patient walks, sits, rises, takes off garments, and responds to directions.

TECHNIQUE	FINDINGS
Inspect skeleton and extremities, comparing sides	
Inspect anterior, posterior, and lateral aspects of posture; ability to stand erect; body parts; and extremities.	
♦ Size, alignment, contour, and symmetry Measure the extremities when lack of symmetry is noted in length or circumference	**Expected:** Bilateral symmetry of length, circumference, alignment, and position and number of skin folds; symmetric body parts; and aligned extremities. *Unexpected:* Gross deformity, lordosis, kyphosis, scoliosis, bony enlargement.

TECHNIQUE	FINDINGS
Inspect skin and subcutaneous tissues over muscles, cartilage, bones, and joints	*Unexpected:* Discoloration, swelling, or masses.
Inspect muscles and compare sides	
♦ Size and symmetry	Expected: Approximately symmetric bilateral muscle size. *Unexpected:* Gross hypertrophy or atrophy, fasciculations, or spasms.
Palpate all bones, joints, and surrounding muscles	
♦ Muscle tone	Expected: Firm. *Unexpected:* Hard or doughy.
♦ Characteristics	*Unexpected:* Heat, tenderness, swelling, crepitus, resistance to pressure, or discomfort to pressure on bones and joints.
Test each major joint and related muscle groups for active and passive range of motion, and compare sides	
Ask patient to move each joint through range of motion (see instructions for specific joints and muscles in individual sections that follow), then ask patient to relax as you passively move same joints until end of range is felt.	Expected: Range of motion equal for each joint and on both sides during both active and passive maneuvers.

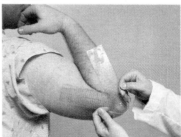

TECHNIQUE	FINDINGS
	Unexpected: Pain, limitation of motion, spastic movement, joint instability, deformity, contracture, crepitation, tenderness, and discrepancies between active and passive range of motion. When increase or limitation in range of motion is found, measure angles of greatest flexion and extension with goniometer, as shown in the figure on p. 158, and compare with values as described for specific joints in individual sections.

MUSCLE STRENGTH

	Scales		
Muscle function level	Grade	% Normal	Lovett scale
No evidence of contractility	0	0	0 (zero)
Slight contractility, no movement	1	10	T (trace)
Full range of motion, gravity eliminated*	2	25	P (poor)
Full range of motion with gravity	3	50	F (fair)
Full range of motion against gravity, some resistance	4	75	G (good)
Full range of motion against gravity, full resistance	5	100	N (normal)

From Barkauskas et al, 1994.
*Passive movement.

TECHNIQUE	FINDINGS

Test major muscle groups for strength and compare contralateral sides

For each muscle group, ask patient to flex muscle and resist as you apply opposing force. Compare bilaterally.

Expected: Bilaterally symmetric with full resistance to opposition. *Unexpected: Inability to produce full resistance. Grade muscular strength according to the table on p. 159.*

Temporomandibular Joint
Palpate joint space for clicking, popping, and pain

Locate temporomandibular joints with fingertips placed just anterior to tragus of each ear, as shown in the figure at right. Ask patient to open mouth and allow fingertips to slip into joint space. Gently palpate.

Expected: Audible or palpable snapping or clicking.
Unexpected: Pain, crepitus, locking, or popping.

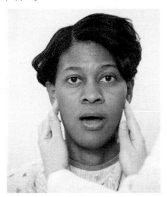

Test range of motion

Ask patient to:
♦ Open and close mouth

♦ Move jaw laterally to each side

Expected: Opens 3 to 6 cm between upper and lower teeth.
Expected: Mandible moves 1 to 2 cm in each direction.

TECHNIQUE	FINDINGS
◆ Protrude and retract jaw	**Expected:** Both protrusion and retraction possible.

Test strength of temporalis muscles with patient's teeth clenched

Ask patient to clench teeth while you palpate contracted muscles and apply opposing force. (This also tests cranial nerve V motor function.)

Expected: Bilaterally symmetric with full resistance to opposition. *Unexpected: Inability to produce full resistance.*

Cervical Spine
Inspect neck

Inspect from anterior and posterior position.
◆ Alignment

Expected: Cervical spine straight, with head erect and in approximate alignment.

◆ Symmetry of skin folds

Unexpected: Asymmetric skin folds.

Palpate posterior neck, cervical spine, and paravertebral, trapezius, and sternocleidomastoid muscles

Expected: Good muscle tone, symmetry in size. *Unexpected: Palpable tenderness or muscle spasm.*

Test range of motion

◆ Forward flexion
Bend head forward, chin to chest.

Expected: 45-degree flexion.

◆ Hyperextension
Bend head backward, chin toward ceiling.

Expected: 45-degree hyperextension.

TECHNIQUE	FINDINGS

♦ Lateral bending
    Bend head to each side, ear to each shoulder.

Expected: 40-degree lateral bending.

♦ Rotation
    Turn head to each side, chin to shoulder.

Expected: 70-degree rotation.

Test strength of sternocleidomastoid and trapezius muscles

Ask patient to maintain each of the previous positions while you apply opposing force. (This also tests cranial nerve XI with rotation.)

Expected: Bilaterally symmetric with full resistance to opposition.
Unexpected: *Inability to produce full resistance.*

Thoracic and Lumbar Spine
Inspect spine for alignment

Note major landmarks of back: each spinal process of vertebrae (C7 and T1 usually most prominent), scapulae, iliac crests, and paravertebral muscles.

Expected: Head positioned directly over gluteal cleft, vertebrae straight (as indicated by symmetric shoulder, scapular, and iliac crest heights), curves of cervical and lumbar spines concave, curve of thoracic spine convex, and knees and feet aligned with trunk and pointing directly forward.
Unexpected: *Lordosis, kyphosis, or sharp angular deformity (gibbus).*

Palpate spinal processes and paravertebral muscles

Ask patient to stand erect.

Unexpected: *Muscle spasm or spinal tenderness.*

TECHNIQUE	FINDINGS

Percuss for spinal tenderness

Patient is still standing erect. First tap each spinal process with one finger, then rap each side of the spine along paravertebral muscles with ulnar aspect of fist.

Unexpected: *Muscle spasm or spinal tenderness.*

Test range of motion and curvature

Ask patient to perform following movements (mark each spinal process with skin pencil if unexpected curvature suspected):

♦ Forward flexion
Bend forward at waist and try to touch toes. Observe from behind to check curvature.

Expected: 75- to 90-degree flexion, with back remaining symmetric as concave curve of lumbar spine becomes convex with forward flexion. **Unexpected:** *Lateral curvature or rib hump.*

♦ Hyperextension
Bend back at waist as far as possible.

Expected: 30-degree hyperextension with reversal of lumbar curve.

♦ Lateral bending
Bend to each side as far as possible.

Expected: 35-degree lateral bending, each side.

♦ Rotation
Swing upper trunk from waist in circular motion front to side to back to side while you stabilize pelvis.

Expected: 30-degree rotation forward and backward.

TECHNIQUE	FINDINGS

Shoulders

Inspect shoulders, shoulder girdle, clavicles and scapulae, and area muscles

♦ Size and contour

Expected: All shoulder structures symmetric in size and contour.
Unexpected: *Asymmetry, hollows in rounding contour, or winged scapula.*

Palpate sternoclavicular and acromioclavicular joints, clavicle, scapulae, coracoid process, greater trochanter of humerus, biceps groove, and area muscles

Expected: No tenderness or masses, bilateral symmetry.
Unexpected: *Pain, tenderness, mass.*

Test range of motion

Ask patient to perform following movements:

♦ Shrugging shoulders
Shrug shoulders.

Expected: Symmetric rising.

♦ Forward flexion
Raise both arms forward and straight up over head.

Expected: 180-degree forward flexion.

♦ Hyperextension
Extend and stretch both arms behind back.

Expected: 50-degree hyperextension.

♦ Abduction
Lift both arms laterally and straight up over head.

Expected: 180-degree abduction.

♦ Adduction
Swing each arm across the front of the body.

Expected: 50-degree adduction.

TECHNIQUE	FINDINGS

♦ Internal rotation
Place both arms be-
hind hips, elbows out.

♦ External
Place both arms be-
hind head, elbows out.

Expected: 90-degree internal rotation.
Expected: 90-degree external rotation.

**Test shoulder girdle
muscle strength**

Ask patient to main-
tain following posi-
tions while you apply
opposing force:

♦ Shrugged shoulders
(This also tests cranial
nerve XI.)

Expected: Bilaterally symmetric
with full resistance to opposition.
*Unexpected: Inability to produce full
resistance.*

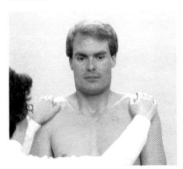

♦ Forward flexion

Expected: Bilaterally symmetric
with full resistance to opposition.
*Unexpected: Inability to produce full
resistance.*

♦ Abduction

Expected: Bilaterally symmetric
with full resistance to opposition.
*Unexpected: Inability to produce full
resistance.*

TECHNIQUE	FINDINGS

Elbows
**Inspect elbows in flexed
and extended positions**

♦ Contour

*Unexpected: Subcutaneous nodules
along pressure points of extensor surface of
ulna.*

♦ Carrying angle
Inspect with arm pas-
sively extended, palm
forward.

Expected: Usually 5 to 15 degrees
laterally.
*Unexpected: Lateral angle exceeding 15
degrees (cubitus valgus) or medial
carrying angle (cubitus varus).*

**Palpate extensor surface
of ulna, olecranon
process, medial and
lateral epicondyles of
humerus, and groove on
each side of olecranon
process**

Palpate with patient's
elbow at 70 degrees.

*Unexpected: Boggy, soft, or fluctuant
swelling; point tenderness at lateral
epicondyle or along grooves of olecranon
process and epicondyles.*

Test range of motion

Ask patient to perform
following movements:
♦ Flexion and extension
Bend and straighten
elbow.

Expected: 160-degree flexion and
180-degree extension.

TECHNIQUE	FINDINGS
◆ Pronation and supination With elbow flexed at right angle, rotate hand from palm side down to palm side up.	**Expected:** 90-degree pronation and 90-degree supination. *Unexpected: Increased pain with pronation and supination of elbow; or tenderness, swelling, and thickening of synovial membrane.*
Test muscle strength Ask patient to maintain flexion and extension, as well as pronation and supination, while you apply opposing force.	**Expected:** Bilaterally symmetric with full resistance to opposition. *Unexpected: Inability to produce full resistance.*

Hands and Wrists
Inspect dorsum and palm of each hand

◆ Characteristics and contour	**Expected:** Palmar and phalangeal creases. Palmar surfaces with central depression with prominent, rounded mound on thumb side (thenar eminence) and less prominent hypothenar eminence on little finger side.
◆ Position	**Expected:** Fingers able to fully extend and be aligned with forearm when in close approximation to each other. *Unexpected: Deviation of fingers to ulnar side or swan-neck or boutonnière deformities.*
◆ Shape	**Expected:** Lateral finger surfaces gradually tapered from proximal to distal aspects.

TECHNIQUE   **FINDINGS**

Palpate each joint in hand and wrist

Palpate interpha-
langeal joints with
thumb and index fin-
ger, as shown in the
figure at right; meta-
carpophalangeal
joints with both
thumbs, as shown in
the figure below, left;
and wrist and radio-
carpal groove with
thumbs on dorsal sur-
face and fingers on
palmar aspect of wrist,
as shown in the figure
below, right.

Expected: Joint surfaces smooth.
Unexpected: *Nodules, swelling,
bogginess, tenderness, or ganglion.*

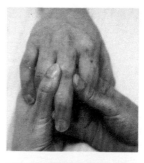

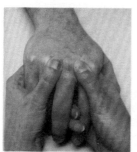 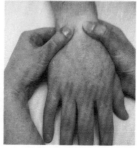

TECHNIQUE	FINDINGS

Strike median nerve for Tinel sign

Strike median nerve where it passes through carpal tunnel with index finger.

Unexpected: *Tingling sensation radiating from wrist to hand along median nerve.*

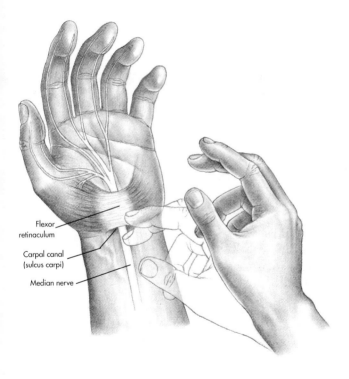

Flexor retinaculum

Carpal canal (sulcus carpi)

Median nerve

TECHNIQUE	FINDINGS

Test range of motion

Ask patient to perform
the following move-
ments:

♦ Metacarpophalangeal
  flexion and hyperex-
  tension
  Bend fingers forward
  at metacarpopha-
  langeal joint, then
  stretch fingers up and
  back at knuckle.

Expected: 90-degree metacarpophalangeal flexion and as much
as 20-degree hyperextension.

♦ Thumb opposition
  Touch thumb to each
  fingertip and to base
  of little finger, then
  make a fist.

Expected: Able to perform all
movements.

♦ Finger abduction and
  adduction
  Spread fingers apart
  and then touch them
  together.

Expected: Both movements possible.

♦ Wrist extension and
  hyperextension
  Bend hand at wrist up
  and down.

Expected: 90-degree flexion and
70-degree hyperextension.

♦ Radial and ulnar mo-
  tion
  With palm side down,
  turn each hand to
  right and left.

Expected: 20-degree radial motion
and 55-degree ulnar motion.

TECHNIQUE	FINDINGS

Test muscle strength

Ask patient to perform following movements:

♦ Wrist extension and hyperextension
Maintain wrist flexion while you apply opposing force.

Expected: Bilaterally symmetric with full resistance to opposition. *Unexpected: Inability to produce full resistance.*

♦ Hand strength
Grip two of your fingers tightly.

Expected: Firm, sustained grip. **Unexpected:** *Weakness or pain.*

Hips

Inspect hips for symmetry and level of gluteal folds

With patient standing, inspect anteriorly and posteriorly, using major landmarks of iliac crest and greater trochanter of femur.

Unexpected: Asymmetry in iliac crest height, size of buttocks, or number and level of gluteal folds.

Palpate hips and pelvis

Have patient lie supine.

Unexpected: Instability, tenderness, or crepitus.

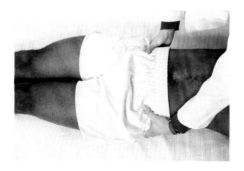

TECHNIQUE	FINDINGS

Test range of motion

While in position indicated, patient should perform following movements:

♦ Flexion, knee extended. With patient supine, raise leg over body.

Expected: Up to 90-degree flexion.

♦ Hyperextension While standing or prone, swing straightened leg behind body.

Expected: Up to 30-degree hyperextension.

♦ Flexion, knee flexed While supine, raise one knee to chest while keeping other leg straight.

Expected: 120-degree flexion.

♦ Abduction and adduction While supine, swing leg laterally and medially with knee straight. During adduction movement, lift patient's opposite leg to permit examined leg full movement.

Expected: Up to 45-degree abduction and up to 30-degree adduction.

♦ Internal rotation While supine, flex knee and rotate leg inward toward other leg.

Expected: 40-degree internal rotation.

♦ External rotation While supine, place lateral aspect of foot on knee of other leg. Move flexed leg toward table.

Expected: 45-degree external rotation.

TECHNIQUE	FINDINGS

Test muscle strength

♦ Knee in flexion and extension
Ask patient to maintain flexion of hip with knee in flexion and then extension while applying opposing force.

Expected: Bilaterally symmetric with full resistance to opposition.
Unexpected: Inability to produce full resistance.

Perform Thomas test to inspect for flexion contractures

While supine, patient should fully extend one leg flat on examining table and flex other leg with knee to chest.

Expected: Patient able to keep extended leg flat on table.
Unexpected: Extended leg lifts off table.

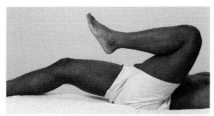

Perform Trendelenburg test to inspect for hip dislocation

Ask patient to stand and balance first on one foot, then the other. Observe from behind.

Unexpected: Asymmetry of iliac crests.

TECHNIQUE	FINDINGS

Legs and Knees

Inspect knees and popliteal spaces, flexed and extended

Note major landmarks: tibial tuberosity, medial and lateral tibial condyles, medial and lateral epicondyles of femur, adductor tubercle of femur, and patella.

Expected: Natural concavities on anterior aspect, on each side, and above patella.

Observe lower leg alignment

Expected: Angle between femur and tibia less than 15 degrees. Bowlegs is a common finding until 18 months of age; knock knees is common between 2 and 4 years. *Unexpected: Knock knees (genu valgum), bowlegs (genu varum), and excessive hyperextension of knee with weight bearing (genu recurvatum).*

Palpate popliteal space

Unexpected: Swelling or tenderness.

Palpate tibiofemoral joint space

Identify patella, suprapatellar pouch, and infrapatellar fat pad.

Expected: Smooth and firm.
Unexpected: Tenderness, bogginess, nodules, or crepitus.

Test range of motion

♦ Flexion
Ask patient to bend each knee.

Expected: 130-degree flexion.

♦ Extension
Ask patient to straighten leg and stretch it.

Expected: Full extension and up to 15-degree hyperextension.

TECHNIQUE	FINDINGS

Test muscle strength

♦ Flexion and extension
Ask patient to maintain flexion and extension while you apply opposing force.

Expected: Bilaterally symmetric with full resistance to opposition.
Unexpected: Inability to produce full resistance.

Additional Techniques for Knees

Perform ballottement procedure to determine presence of excess fluid or an effusion in knee

With knee extended, apply downward pressure on suprapatellar pouch with thumb and fingers of one hand, then push the patella sharply backward against femur with finger of other hand, as shown at right. Suddenly release pressure on patella, while keeping finger lightly on knee.

Unexpected: A "tap" against finger after releasing pressure.

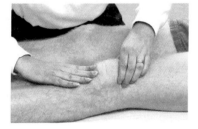

TECHNIQUE	FINDINGS

Test for bulge sign to determine presence of excess fluid in knee

With knee extended, milk medial aspect of knee upward two or three times, as shown below, then tap lateral side of patella, as shown below, right.

Unexpected: Bulge of returning fluid to hollow area medial to patella.

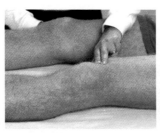
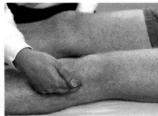

Perform McMurray test to detect torn meniscus

Ask patient to lie supine and flex one knee completely with foot flat on table near buttocks. Maintain that flexion with your thumb and index finger, while stabilizing knee. Hold heel with other hand, rotate foot and lower leg to lateral position, and extend knee to 90-degree angle.

Return knee to full flexion, then rotate foot and lower leg to

Unexpected: Palpable or audible click or limited extension of knee with either procedure.

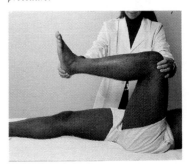

TECHNIQUE	FINDINGS

medial position, and
extend knee to 90-de-
gree angle.

**Perform drawer test to
identify instability of knee**

♦ Medial and lateral sta-
bility
Ask patient to lie
supine and extend
knee. While you stabi-
lize femur with one
hand and hold ankle
with other, try to
abduct and adduct
knee.

Unexpected: *Medial or lateral movement.*

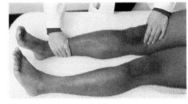

♦ Anterior and posterior
stability
Ask patient to flex
knee 90 degrees, plac-
ing foot flat on table.
While stabilizing foot
with one hand and
grasping lower leg just
below knee with other,
try to push lower leg
forward and pull back-
ward.

Unexpected: *Anterior or posterior movement.*

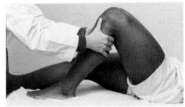

**Perform Apley test to
detect torn meniscus**

Ask patient to lie
prone and flex knee to
90 degrees. Place
hand on heel of foot
and press firmly, op-
posing tibia to femur.
Carefully rotate lower
leg externally and in-
ternally.

Unexpected: *Clicks, locking, or pain.*

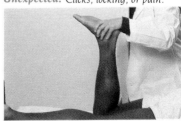

TECHNIQUE	FINDINGS

Feet and Ankles

Inspect during weight bearing (standing and walking) and nonweight bearing

Note major landmarks: medial malleolus, lateral malleolus, and Achilles tendon.

♦ Characteristics

Expected: Smooth and rounded malleolar prominence, prominent heels, and prominent metatarsophalangeal joints.
Unexpected: Calluses and corns.

♦ Alignment

Expected: Feet aligned with tibias and weight bearing on foot midline.
Unexpected: In-toeing (pes varus), out-toeing (pes valgus), deviations in forefoot alignment (metatarsus varus or metatarsus valgus), heel pronation, or pain.

♦ Contour

Expected: Longitudinal arch that may flatten with weight bearing. Foot flat when not bearing weight (pes planus) and high instep (pes cavus) are common variations.
Unexpected: Pain with pes planus.

♦ Toes

Expected: Toes on each foot straight forward, flat, and in alignment.
Unexpected: Hammer toe; claw toe; hallux valgus; bunions, or heat, redness, swelling, and tenderness of the metatarsophalangeal joint of great toe (possibly with draining tophus).

TECHNIQUE	FINDINGS

Palpate Achilles tendon and each metatarsal joint

Using thumb and fingers of both hands, compress forefoot, palpating each metatarsophalangeal joint.

Expected: No tenderness or masses, bilateral symmetry.
Unexpected: Pain, *masses*.

Test range of motion

Ask patient to sit then perform following movements:

♦ Dorsiflexion
Point foot toward ceiling.

Expected: 20-degree dorsiflexion.

♦ Plantar flexion
Point foot toward floor.

Expected: 45-degree plantar flexion.

♦ Inversion and eversion
Bend foot at ankle, then turn sole of foot toward and away from other foot.

Expected: 30-degree inversion and 20-degree eversion.

♦ Abduction and adduction
Rotate ankle, turning away from and then toward other foot (while you stabilize leg).

Expected: 10-degree abduction and 20-degree adduction.

♦ Flexion and extension
Bend and straighten toes.

Expected: Some flexion and extension, especially great toes.

TECHNIQUE	FINDINGS
Test strength of ankle muscles	
Ask patient to maintain dorsiflexion and plantar flexion while you apply opposing force.	**Expected:** Bilaterally symmetric with full resistance to opposition. **Unexpected:** *Inability to produce full resistance.*

Children

Test for Gower sign in children	
Observe the child at play and evaluate gross motor skills to obtain a sense of muscle strength.	**Expected:** Ability to rise to a standing position from a supine position without using arms for leverage. **Unexpected:** *Child rises from a sitting position by placing hands on legs and pushing trunk up.*

AIDS TO DIFFERENTIAL DIAGNOSIS

ABNORMALITY	DESCRIPTION
Carpal tunnel syndrome	Numbness, burning, and tingling in hands, often occurring at night but also elicited by rotational movement of wrist. Pain in arms. Can result in weakness of hand and flattening of the thenar eminence of palm.
Gout	Red, hot, swollen joint (classically the proximal phalanx of great toe, although other joints of wrist, hands, ankles, and knees are sometimes affected); exquisite pain; limited range of motion; tophi; and mild fever.

DIFFERENTIAL DIAGNOSIS OF ARTHRITIS

Signs and symptoms	Osteoarthritis	Rheumatoid arthritis
Onset	Insidious	Gradual or sudden (24-48 hr)
Duration of stiffness	Few minutes, localized, but short "gelling" after prolonged rest	Often hours, most pronounced after rest
Pain	On motion, with prolonged activity, relieved by rest	Even at rest, may disturb sleep
Weakness	Usually localized and not severe	Often pronounced, out of proportion with muscle atrophy
Fatigue	Unusual	Often severe, with onset 4-5 hr after rising
Emotional depression and lability	Unusual	Common, coincides with fatigue and disease activity, often relieved if in remission
Tenderness localized over afflicted joint	Common	Almost always, most sensitive indicator of inflammation
Swelling	Effusion common, little synovial reaction	Fusiform soft tissue enlargement, effusion common, synovial proliferation and thickening
Heat, erythema	Unusual	Sometimes present
Crepitus, crackling	Coarse to medium on motion	Medium to fine
Joint enlargement	Mild with firm consistency	Moderate to severe

Modified from McCarty, 1993.

ABNORMALITY	DESCRIPTION
Bursitis	Motion limitation caused by swelling, pain on movement, point tenderness, erythema, and warmth; commonly occurs in shoulder, elbow, hip, and knee.
Osteoarthritis	See the table on p. 181.
Rheumatoid arthritis	See the table on p. 181.
Sprain	Pain, marked swelling, hemorrhage, and loss of function.
Fracture	Deformity, edema, pain, loss of function, color changes, and paresthesia.
Tenosynovitis	Point tenderness, edema, pain with movement, and weakness, commonly of shoulder, knee, heel, and wrist.
Scoliosis	Uneven shoulder and hip levels, a rib hump, and flank asymmetry on forward flexion. Lateral curvature of spine resulting from leg length discrepancy also possible.
Osteoporosis	Height loss, bent spine, and the appearance of sinking into hips—most often in postmenopausal women. Usual presenting symptom is acute, painful fracture, most commonly of hip, vertebra, or wrist.

SAMPLE DOCUMENTATION

Posture straight, without scoliosis; muscles and extremities symmetric; muscle strength appropriate and equal bilaterally; active range of motion without pain or limitation in all joints except right knee; clicks, pain, locking, and limited extension noted with Apley and McMurray tests.

Neurologic System and Mental Status

EQUIPMENT

♦ Familiar objects (coins, keys, paper clip)
♦ Vials of aromatic substances (coffee, orange, peppermint, banana)
♦ Sterile needles
♦ Cotton wisp
♦ Tongue blades (one intact and one broken with point and rounded edges)
♦ List of tastes
♦ Vials of solutions (glucose, salt, lemon or vinegar, and quinine) with applicators
♦ Cup of water
♦ Test tubes of hot and cold water
♦ Tuning forks
♦ Reflex hammer

EXAMINATION

Evaluate the neurologic system as the rest of the body is examined. Assessment of mental state is implicit in taking a routine history. When history and examination findings have not re-

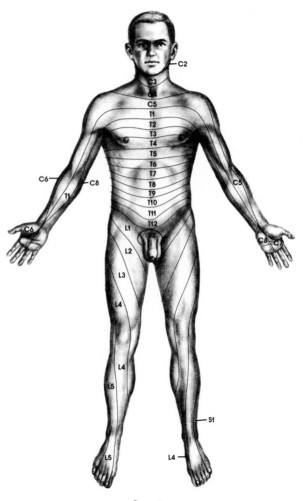

Dermatomes

vealed a potential neurologic problem, perform a neurologic screening examination as shown in the box on p. 186, rather than a full neurologic examination. See Chapter 14, Musculoskeletal System, for evaluation of muscle tone and strength.

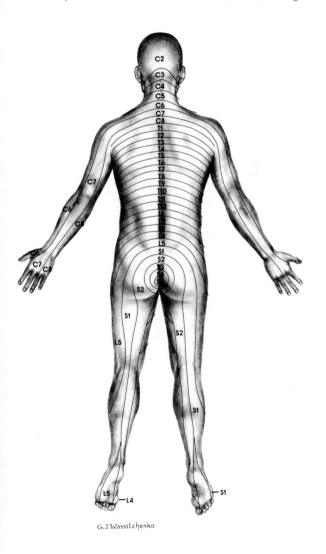

G.J.Wassilchenko

NEUROLOGIC SCREENING EXAMINATION

This shorter screening examination is commonly used for health visits when no known neurologic problem is apparent.

Mental status

Information is generally obtained during the history in the following areas:

Appearance
Grooming
Emotional status
Body language

Emotional stability
Mood and feelings
Thought processes

Cognitive abilities
State of consciousness
Memory
Attention span
Judgment

Speech and language
Voice quality
Articulation
Comprehension
Coherence
Aphasia

Cranial nerves

Cranial nerves II through XII are routinely tested; however, taste and smell are not tested unless some aberration is found.

Proprioception and cerebellar function

One test is administered for each of the following: rapid rhythmic alternating movements, accuracy of movements, balance (Romberg test), and gait and heel-toe walking.

Sensory function

Superficial pain and touch at a distal point in each extremity are tested; vibration and position senses are assessed by testing the great toe.

Deep tendon reflexes

All deep tendon reflexes are tested, excluding the test for clonus.

TECHNIQUE	FINDINGS

Mental Status and Speech Patterns
Observe physical appearance and behavior

♦ Grooming

Unexpected: *Poor hygiene, lack of concern with appearance, or inappropriate dress for season, gender, or occasion in previously well-groomed patient.*

♦ Emotional status

Expected: Patient expressing concern with visit appropriate for emotional content of topics discussed.
Unexpected: *Behavior conveying carelessness, indifference, inability to sense emotions in others, loss of sympathetic reactions, unusual docility, rage reactions, or excessive irritability.*

♦ Body language

Expected: Erect posture and eye contact.
Unexpected: *Slumped posture, lack of facial expression, excessively energetic movements, or constantly watchful eyes.*

Investigate cognitive abilities

The Mini-Mental State Examination may be used to quantitatively estimate cognitive function or document changes. (See p. 188.)

♦ State of consciousness

Expected: Oriented to time, place, and person, and able to appropriately respond to questions and environmental stimuli.
Unexpected: *See the box on p. 189.*

Patient.................................
Examiner.................................
Date ....

"MINI-MENTAL STATE"

Maximum
Score   Score

ORIENTATION

5   ( )   What is the (year) (season) (date) (day) (month)?
5   ( )   Where are we: (state) (county) (town) (hospital) (floor).

REGISTRATION

3   ( )   Name 3 objects: 1 second to say each. Then ask the patient all 3 after you have said them. Give 1 point for each correct answer. Then repeat them until he learns all 3. Count trials and record.
            Trials

ATTENTION AND CALCULATION

5   ( )   Serial 7's. 1 point for each correct. Stop after 5 answers. Alternatively spell "world" backwards.

RECALL

3   ( )   Ask for the 3 objects repeated above. Give 1 point for each correct.

LANGUAGE

9   ( )   Name a pencil, and watch (2 points)
            Repeat the following "No ifs, ands or buts." (1 point)
            Follow a 3-stage command:
                "Take a paper in your right hand, fold it in half, and put in on the floor" (3 points)
            Read and obey the following:
            CLOSE YOUR EYES (1 point)
            Write a sentence (1 point)
            Copy design (1 point)
_____   Total score
            ASSESS level of consciousness along a continuum_____
                                        Alert   Drowsy   Stupor   Coma

INSTRUCTIONS FOR ADMINISTRATION OF
MINI-MENTAL STATE EXAMINATION

ORIENTATION

(1) Ask for the date. Then ask specifically for parts omitted, e.g., "Can you also tell me what season it is?" One point for each correct.
(2) Ask in turn "Can you tell me the name of this hospital?" (town, county, etc.). One point for each correct.

REGISTRATION

Ask the patient if you may test his memory. Then say the name of 3 unrelated objects, clearly and slowly, about one second for each. After you have said all 3, ask him to repeat them. The first repetition determines his score (0-3) but keep saying them until he can repeat all 3, up to 6 trials. If he does not eventually learn all 3, recall cannot be meaningfully tested.

ATTENTION AND CALCULATION

Ask the patient to begin with 100 and count backwards by 7. Stop after 5 subtractions (93,86,79,72,65). Score the total number of correct answers.
If the patient cannot or will not perform this task, ask him to spell the word "world" backwards. The score is the number of letters in correct order. E.g. dlrow = 5, dlorw = 3.

RECALL

Ask the patient if he can recall the 3 words you previously asked him to remember. Score 0-3.

LANGUAGE

Naming: Show the patient a wrist watch and ask him what it is. Repeat for pencil. Score 0-2.
Repetition: Ask the patient to repeat the sentence after you. Allow only one trial. Score 0 or 1.
3-Stage command: Give the patient a piece of plain blank paper and repeat the command. Score 1 point for each part correctly executed.
Reading: On a blank piece of paper print the sentence "Close your eyes", in letters large enough for the patient to see clearly. Ask him to read it and do what it says. Score 1 point only if he actually closes his eyes.
Writing: Give the patient a blank piece of paper and ask him to write a sentence for you. Do not dictate a sentence, it is to be written spontaneously. It must contain a subject and verb to be sensible. Correct grammar and punucation are not necessary.
Copying: On a clean piece of paper, draw intersecting pentagons, each side about 1 in., and ask him to copy it exactly as it is. All 10 angles must be present and 2 must intersect to score 1 point. Tremor and rotation are ignored.
Estimate the patient's level of sensorium along a continuum, from alert on the left to coma on the right.

UNEXPECTED LEVELS OF CONSCIOUSNESS

CONFUSION	Inappropriate response to question
	Decreased attention span and memory
LETHARGY	Drowsy, falls asleep quickly
	Once aroused, responds appropriately
DELIRIUM	Confusion with disordered perceptions and decreased attention span
	Marked anxiety with motor and sensory excitement
	Inappropriate reactions to stimuli
STUPOR	Arousable for short periods to visual, verbal, or painful stimuli
	Simple motor or moaning responses to stimuli
	Slow responses
COMA	Neither awake nor aware
	Decerebrate posturing to painful stimuli

TECHNIQUE	FINDINGS
♦ Analogies Ask patient to describe analogies, first simple, then more complex:	*Unexpected*: *Inability to describe similarities or differences.*
♦ What is similar about peaches and lemons, oceans and lakes, pencils and typewriters?	
♦ An engine is to an airplane as an oar is to a _____?	
♦ What is different about a magazine and a telephone book, and bush and tree?	

TECHNIQUE	FINDINGS
♦ Abstract reasoning	
Ask patient to explain meaning of fable, proverb, or metaphor:	**Unexpected:** *Inability to give adequate explanation.*
♦ A stitch in time saves nine.	
♦ A bird in the hand is worth two in a bush.	
♦ A rolling stone gathers no moss.	
♦ Arithmetic calculations	
Ask patient to perform simple calculations without paper:	**Unexpected:** *Inability to complete with few errors within a minute.*
♦ 50 – 7, –7, –7, etc., until the answer is 8.	
♦ 50 + 8, +8, +8. etc., until the answer is 98.	
♦ Writing ability	
Ask patient to write name and address or a phrase you dictate (or draw simple figures—triangle, circle, square, flower, house—if unable to write).	**Unexpected:** *Omission or addition of letters, syllables, or words; mirror writing; or uncoordinated writing (or drawing for patients unable to write).*
♦ Execution of motor skills	
Ask patient to do a motor task such as combing hair.	**Unexpected:** *Inability to complete a task.*

TECHNIQUE	FINDINGS

♦ Memory

Immediate recall: Ask patient to listen to, then repeat, a sentence or series of numbers (5 to 8 numbers forward, 4 to 6 numbers backward).

Expected:
Immediate recall: Able to repeat sentence or numbers.
Recent memory: Able to remember test objects.
Remote memory: Able to recall verifiable past events.
Unexpected: *Impaired memory.*

Recent memory: Show patient three or four objects, and say you will ask about them later. In 10 minutes, ask patient to list objects.

Remote memory: Ask patient about verifiable past events (e.g., mother's maiden name, name of high school).

♦ Attention span

Unexpected: *Easy distraction or confusion, negativism.*

♦ Judgment
Explore:
  ♦ How patient meets social and family obligations; patient's future plans.
  ♦ Patient's solutions to hypothetical situations (e.g., found stamped envelope or was stopped for running a red light).

Expected: Ability to evaluate situation and provide appropriate response.

TECHNIQUE	FINDINGS

♦ Patient's explanation to fables (e.g., "The Tortoise and the Hare") or metaphors.

Evaluate emotional stability

♦ Mood and feelings
Ask patient how he or she feels, if feelings are a problem in daily life, and if he or she has particularly difficult times or experiences.

Expected: Appropriate feelings for the situation.
Unexpected: Unresponsiveness, hopelessness, agitation, euphoria, irritability, or wide mood swings.

♦ Thought process and content
Ask patient about obsessive thought content and obsessive behavior.

Expected: Appropriate sequence, logic, coherence, and relevance to topics discussed.
Unexpected: Illogical or unrealistic thought process, blocking, or disturbance in stream of thinking. Obsessive thought content or behavior that interferes with daily life or is disabling.

♦ Perceptual distortions and hallucinations
Ask patient about any sensations not believed caused by external stimuli.

Unexpected: Auditory, visual, or tactile hallucinations: hears voices, sees vivid images or shadowy figures, smells offensive odors, feels worms crawling on skin.

Observe speech and language

♦ Voice quality

Expected: Patient uses inflections, speaks clearly and strongly, and is able to increase voice volume.

TECHNIQUE	FINDINGS
♦ Articulation	*Unexpected: Difficulty or discomfort making laryngeal speech sounds.* **Expected:** Proper pronunciation, fluent, and rhythmic, with clear expression of thought. *Unexpected: Imperfect pronunciation, difficulty articulating single speech sound, rapid-fire delivery, or speech with hesitancy, stuttering, repetitions, or slow utterances.*
♦ Comprehension	**Expected:** Able to follow simple instructions.
♦ Coherence	**Expected:** Patient's intentions or perceptions clearly conveyed. *Unexpected: Circumlocutions, perseveration, disorderly words or sentences, gibberish, neologisms, echolalia, or unusual sounds.*
♦ Ability to communicate	*Unexpected: Hesitations, omissions, inappropriate word substitutions, circumlocutions, neologisms, disturbance of rhythm or words in sequence or other signs of aphasia.*

Cranial Nerves I-XII

The table on pp. 194-195 summarizes the cranial nerve examination.

Assess olfactory nerve (CN I)

Ask patient to close eyes. Occlude one naris, hold vial under nose, and ask patient to breathe deeply and identify odor. Allow patient to breathe comfortably, then occlude other naris and

Expected: Able to perceive and usually identify odor on each side.
Unexpected: Anosmia.

PROCEDURES FOR CRANIAL NERVE EXAMINATION

Cranial nerve (CN)	Procedure
CN I (Olfactory)	Test ability to identify familiar aromatic odors, one naris at a time with eyes closed.
CN II (Optic)	Test vision with Snellen chart and Rosenbaum near vision chart. Perform ophthalmoscopic examination of fundi. Test visual fields by confrontation and extinction of vision.
CN III, IV, and VI (Oculomotor, tro-chlear, and abducens)	Test extraocular movement. Inspect eyelids for drooping. Inspect pupils' size for equality and their direct and consensual response to light and accommodation.
CN V (Trigeminal)	Inspect face for muscle atrophy and tremors. Palpate jaw muscles for tone and strength when patient clenches teeth. Test superficial pain and touch sensation in each branch. (Test temperature sensation if there are unexpected findings to pain or touch.) Test corneal reflex.
CN VII (Facial)	Inspect symmetry of facial features with various expressions (e.g., smile, frown, puffed cheeks, wrinkled forehead). Test ability to identify sweet and salty tastes on each side of tongue.

PROCEDURES FOR CRANIAL NERVE EXAMINATION—cont'd

Cranial nerve (CN)	Procedure
CN VIII (Acoustic)	Test sense of hearing with whisper screening tests or by audiometry. Compare bone and air conduction of sound. Test for lateralization of sound.
CN IX (Glossopharyngeal)	Test ability to identify sour and bitter tastes. Test gag reflex and ability to swallow.
CN X (Vagus)	Inspect palate and uvula for symmetry with speech sounds and gag reflex. Observe for swallowing difficulty. Evaluate quality of guttural speech sounds (presence of nasal or hoarse quality to voice).
CN XI (Spinal accessory)	Test trapezius muscle strength (shrug shoulders against resistance). Test sternocleidomastoid muscle strength (turn head to each side against resistance).
CN XII (Hypoglossal)	Inspect tongue in mouth and while protruded for symmetry, tremors, and atrophy. Inspect tongue movement toward nose and chin. Test tongue strength with index finger when tongue is pressed against cheek. Evaluate quality of lingual speech sounds (*l*, *t*, *d*, *n*).

TECHNIQUE	FINDINGS

repeat with different odor. Continue, alternating two or three odors.

Assess optic nerve (CN II)

See tests for visual acuity and visual fields in Chapter 5, Eyes.

Assess oculomotor, trochlear, and abducens nerves (CN III, CN IV, and CN VI)

See tests for six cardinal points of gaze, pupil size, shape, response to light and accommodation, and opening of upper eyelids in Chapter 5, Eyes.

Unexpected: Absence of lateral gaze. Absence of any expected findings.

Assess trigeminal nerve (CN V)

♦ Facial characteristics

Unexpected: Muscle atrophy, deviation of jaw to one side, or fasciculations.

♦ Muscle tone
Ask patient to clench teeth tightly as you palpate muscles over jaw.

Expected: Symmetric tone.
Unexpected: Fasciculations.

♦ Touch sensation
Ask patient to close eyes and report if sensation to touch is present or is sharp or dull as you touch each side of face at scalp, cheek,

Expected: Symmetric sensory discrimination over face to all stimuli.
Unexpected: Impaired sensation. If impaired, use test tubes of hot and cold water to evaluate temperature sensation.

TECHNIQUE	FINDINGS

and chin areas, alternately using sharp and rounded edges of tongue blades or paper clip, in an unpredictable pattern.
Ask patient to report when the stimulus is felt as you stroke same six areas with cotton wisp or brush. Finally, test sensation over buccal mucosa with wooden applicator.

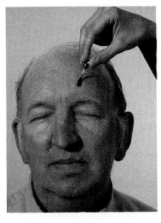

♦ Corneal reflex
   See test for corneal sensitivity in Chapter 5, Eyes.

Unexpected: *Failure to blink.*

Assess facial nerve (CN VII)

♦ Expressions
   Ask patient to make following facial expressions:
   ♦ Raise eyebrows and wrinkle forehead
   ♦ Smile
   ♦ Frown
   ♦ Puff out cheeks
   ♦ Purse lips and blow out
   ♦ Show teeth
   ♦ Squeeze eyes shut

Unexpected: *Tics, unusual facial movements, or asymmetry of expression.*

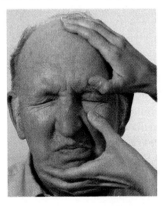

TECHNIQUE	FINDINGS
♦ Speech	**Unexpected:** *Difficulties with enunciating b, m, and p (labial sounds).*
♦ Muscle strength	**Unexpected:** *One side of mouth drooping, flattened nasolabial fold, or lower eyelid sagging.*
♦ Taste (CN VII and CN IX) Hold card listing tastes in patient's view. Ask patient to extend tongue and point to taste as perceived. Apply one of four solutions to lateral side of tongue in appropriate taste-bud region. Offer patient a sip of water and repeat with different solution and applicator, testing each side of tongue with each solution.	**Expected:** Able to identify each taste bilaterally when placed in appropriate taste-bud region.

Assess acoustic nerve (CN VIII)

See screening tests in Chapter 6, Ears, Nose, and Throat.

Assess glossopharyngeal nerve (CN IX)

♦ Taste
See previous information regarding taste.
♦ Gag reflex (nasopharyngeal sensation)
See following step for vagus nerve.

TECHNIQUE	FINDINGS

Assess vagus nerve (CN X)

♦ Gag reflex (nasopharyngeal sensation) (CN IX and CN X)
Tell patient you will be testing gag reflex. Touch posterior wall of pharynx with applicator while observing palate, pharyngeal muscles, and uvula.

Expected: Upward movement of palate and contraction of pharyngeal muscles, with uvula in midline.
Unexpected: Drooping or absence of arch on either side of soft palate.

♦ Motor function
Ask patient to say "ah" while observing movement of soft plate and uvula.

Unexpected: Failure of soft palate to rise or deviation of uvula from midline.

♦ Swallowing (CN IX and CN X)
Ask patient to swallow water.

Expected: Water easily swallowed.
Unexpected: Retrograde passage of water through nose.

♦ Speech

Unexpected: Hoarseness, nasal quality, or difficulty with guttural sounds.

Assess spinal accessory nerve (CN XI)

See Chapter 4, Head and Neck, and Chapter 14, Musculoskeletal System, for evaluations of the size, shape, and strength of the trapezius and sternocleidomastoid muscles.

TECHNIQUE	FINDINGS

Assess hypoglossal nerve (XII)

♦ Tongue resting and protruded
Inspect while at rest on floor of mouth and while protruded.

Unexpected: *Fasciculations, asymmetry, atrophy, or deviation from midline.*

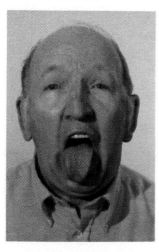

♦ Tongue movement
Ask patient to move tongue in and out, side to side, curled up toward nose, and curled down toward chin.

Expected: Able to perform most tongue movements.

♦ Tongue strength
Ask patient to push tongue against cheek while you apply resistance with index finger.

Expected: Steady, firm pressure.

♦ Speech

Unexpected: *Problems with l, t, d, or n (lingual sounds).*

TECHNIQUE	FINDINGS

Proprioception and Cerebellar Function
Evaluate coordination and fine motor skills

Have patient sit.
♦ Rapid, rhythmic, alternating movements
Ask patient to pat knees with both hands, alternately patting with palms then backs of the hands.

Expected: Smooth execution, maintaining rhythm with increasing speed.
Unexpected: *Stiff, slowed, nonrhythmic, or jerky clonic movements.*

♦ Accuracy of movement: finger-to-finger test
Position your index finger 40 to 50 cm from patient. Ask patient to alternately touch his or her nose and your index finger with the index finger of one hand, as shown at right, while you occasionally change location of your index finger. Repeat with patient's other hand.

Expected: Movements rapid, smooth, and accurate.
Unexpected: *Consistent past pointing.*

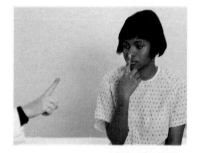

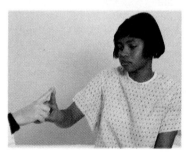

TECHNIQUE	FINDINGS
♦ Accuracy of movement: finger-to-nose test	
Ask patient to close both eyes and touch his or her nose with index finger of each hand while alternating hands and gradually increasing speed.	**Expected:** Movements rapid, smooth, and accurate, even with increasing speed.
♦ Accuracy of movement: heel-to-shin test	
Ask patient to run heel of one foot along shin from knee to ankle of opposite leg. Repeat with other heel. (Also can be performed standing or supine.)	**Expected:** Able to move heel up and down shin in straight line, without irregular deviations to side.

Evaluate balance

♦ Balance: Romberg test	
Ask patient to stand with feet together and arms at sides, first with eyes open, then closed. ***Stand close by in case patient starts to fall.***	**Expected:** Slight swaying movement. *Unexpected: Staggering, losing balance, or swaying to the extent of falling.*
♦ Balance: recovery	
Ask patient to spread feet slightly, then push shoulders to throw her or him off balance. ***Be prepared to catch patient.***	**Expected:** Quick recovery of balance.

TECHNIQUE	FINDINGS
◆ Balance: hopping Have patient hop in place on one foot, then the other, with eyes open.	**Expected:** Able to hop 5 seconds without losing balance. **Unexpected:** *Instability, need to continually touch floor with opposite foot, or tendency to fall.*
◆ Gait: walking Ask patient to walk without shoes around examining room or down hallway, first with eyes open, then closed.	**Expected:** Smooth, regular gait rhythm and symmetric stride length; upright trunk posture swaying with gait phase; and arm swing smooth and symmetric. **Unexpected:** *Shuffling, widely placed feet, toe walking, foot flop, leg lag, scissoring, loss of arm swing, staggering, or reeling.*
◆ Gait: straight-line walking Ask patient to walk a straight line, first forward and then backward, with eyes open and arms at side. Ask patient to touch toe of one foot with heel of other.	**Expected:** Consistent contact between toe and heel with slight swaying. **Unexpected:** *Extension of arms for balance, instability, tendency to fall, or lateral staggering and reeling.*

Sensory Function
Test primary sensory functions

Ask patient to close eyes for all tests. Use minimal stimulation initially, then increase gradually until patient becomes aware. Test contralateral areas, asking patient to compare perceived sensations side to side.	**Expxected:** *For all tests,* minimal differences side to side, correct interpretation of sensations, discrimination of side of body tested, and location of sensation. **Unexpected:** For all tests, *map boundaries of any impairment by distribution of major peripheral nerves or dermatomes (see figures on pp. 184-185).*

Technique	**Findings**

- Superficial touch
  Lightly touch skin with cotton wisp or your fingertips, as shown below. Ask patient to point to area touched or acknowledge when sensation is felt.

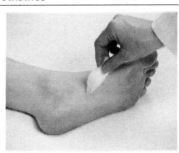

- Superficial pain
  Alternating sharp and smooth edge of broken tongue blade or point and hub of sterile needle, touch skin in unpredictable pattern. Ask patient to identify sensation (sharp or dull) and where it is felt.

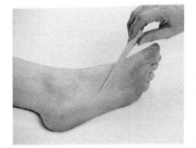

- Temperature and deep pressure
  Necessary to perform test only if superficial pain sensation is not intact.
  Temperature: Alternately roll test tubes of hot and cold water against skin in an unpredictable pattern. Ask patient to indicate hot or cold and where it is felt. Deep pressure: Squeeze trapezius, calf, or biceps muscle.

Expected: Discomfort with deep pressure.

TECHNIQUE	FINDINGS

♦ Vibration

Place stem of vibrating tuning fork against several bony prominences (e.g., toes, ankle, shin, finger joints, wrist, elbow, shoulder, and sternum), beginning distally. Ask patient when and where sensation is felt and what it feels like. Dampen occasionally to see if patient notices difference.

Expected: Buzzing or tingling sensation.

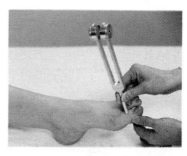

♦ Position of joints

Hold joint to be tested (great toe or finger) by lateral aspects in neutral position, then raise or lower digit, as shown, and ask patient which way it was moved. Return to neutral before moving in another direction. Repeat so both feet and both hands are tested.

Expected: Patient correctly identifies position of joint.

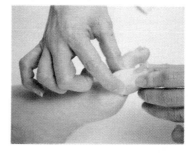

TECHNIQUE	FINDINGS

**Test cortical sensory
functions.**

Ask patient to close
eyes for all tests.

♦ Stereognosis
Hand patient familiar
objects (e.g., key,
coin), and ask patient
to identify.

Unexpected: *Inability to recognize
objects (tactile agnosia).*

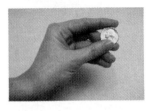

♦ Two-point discrimina-
tion
Using two sterile nee-
dles, alternately touch
patient's skin with one
point or both points
simultaneously at var-
ious locations. Find
distance at which pa-
tient can no longer
distinguish two
points.

Expected: See the table on p. 207.

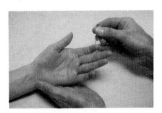

MINIMAL DISTANCES OF DISCRIMINATING TWO POINTS

Body part	Minimal distance (mm)
Tongue	1
Fingertips	2.8
Toes	3-8
Palms of hands	8-12
Chest and forearms	40
Back	40-70
Upper arms and thighs	75

From Barkauskas et al, 1994.

TECHNIQUE	FINDINGS
♦ Extinction phenomenon Simultaneously touch cheek, hand, or other area on each side of body with sterile needle. Ask patient the number of stimuli and locations.	**Expected:** Both sensations felt.
♦ Graphesthesia With blunt pen or applicator stick, draw letter or number on palm of patient's hand, and ask patient to identify it. Repeat with different figure on other hand.	**Expected:** Letter or number readily recognized. 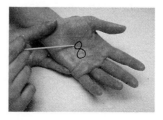

TECHNIQUE	FINDINGS

♦ Point location
Touch area on patient's skin and withdraw stimulus. Ask patient to point to area touched.

Expected: Able to locate stimulus.

Reflexes
Test superficial reflexes

Have patient supine
♦ Abdominal
Stroke each quadrant of abdomen with end of reflex hammer or with tongue blade edge.

Expected: Slight, bilaterally equal movement of umbilicus toward each area of stimulation.

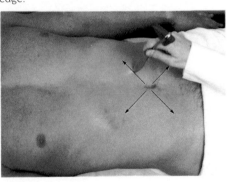

♦ Cremasteric (male patients)
Stroke inner thigh, proximal to distal.

Expected: Testicle and scrotum rise on stroked side.

TECHNIQUE	FINDINGS

◆ Plantar reflex
Using pointed object, stroke lateral side of foot from heel to ball, then curve across ball to medial side.

Expected: Plantar flexion of all toes.
Unexpected: Fanning of toes or dorsiflexion of great toe with or without fanning of other toes (Babinski sign).

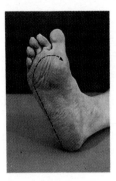

Test deep tendon reflexes

Patient relaxed and either sitting or lying for most procedures. Test each reflex, comparing responses on corresponding sides. Score the deep tendon reflexes on scale shown in the table on p. 210.

Expected: Symmetric visible or palpable responses.
Unexpected: Absent or diminished responses (0 or 1+), or hyperactive reflexes (3+ or 4+). See also the box on p. 210.

◆ Biceps
Flex arm up 45 degrees at elbow, then palpate biceps tendon in antecubital fossa. Place thumb over tendon and fingers over biceps muscle. Strike your thumb with reflex hammer.

Expected: Visible or palpable flexion of elbow.

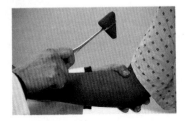

SCORING DEEP TENDON REFLEXES

Grade	Deep tendon reflex response
0	No response
1+	Sluggish or diminished
2+	Active or expected response
3+	More brisk than expected, slightly hyperactive
4+	Brisk, hyperactive, with intermittent or transient clonus

TECHNIQUE   **FINDINGS**

♦ Brachioradial
Flex patient's arm up to 45 degrees while resting patient's forearm on your arm, with hand slightly pronated. Strike brachioradial tendon.

Expected: Pronation of forearm and flexion of elbow.

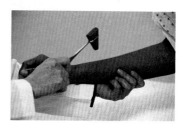

♦ Triceps
Flex patient's arm at elbow up to 90 degrees and rest patient's hand against the side of the body. Palpate triceps tendon and strike directly with reflex hammer, just above elbow.

Expected: Visible or palpable extension of elbow.

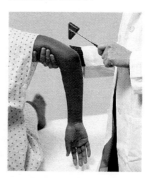

TECHNIQUE	FINDINGS

♦ Patellar
   Flex patient's knee up
   to 90 degrees, allow-
   ing lower leg to hang
   loosely. Support upper
   leg so it does not rest
   against edge of exam-
   ining table, then strike
   patellar tendon just
   below patella.

Expected: Extension of lower leg.

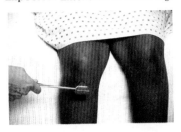

♦ Achilles
   Ask patient to sit.
   Then flex patient's
   knee and dorsiflex an-
   kle up to 90 degrees,
   holding heel of foot.
   Strike Achilles tendon
   at level of ankle malle-
   oli.

Expected: Plantar flexion.

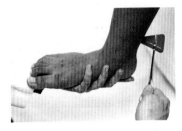

♦ Clonus
   Support patient's knee
   in partially flexed position and briskly dorsiflex the foot with
   other hand, maintain-
   ing foot in flexion.

Unexpected: *Rhythmic oscillating
movements between dorsiflexion and
plantar flexion palpated.*

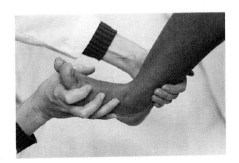

AIDS TO DIFFERENTIAL DIAGNOSIS

ABNORMALITY	DESCRIPTION
Depression	Mood and affect include extreme sadness, anxiety, and agitation. Somatic complaints include altered appetite, constipation, headache, and fatigue.
Dementia	Insidious onset; depressed, apathetic mood persists. Speech may be rambling or incoherent. Memory and thought patterns may be affected. Persistent condition.
Delirium	Sudden onset; this condition lasts for hours or days. Mood and affect include rapid mood swings, fear, and suspicion. Slurred or rapid and manic speech and hallucinations are common. Sleep-wake cycle is disturbed.
AIDS dementia complex (HIV encephalopathy)	Onset (headaches, loss of memory and concentration, and inability to follow complex instructions) leading to global cognitive impairment. Behavior changes include apathy to work, recreation, and social activities. Motor findings include hyperreflexia; increased tone; slowed rapid alternating movements; clumsiness and weakness in arms and legs; and gait ataxia. Possible fecal and urinary incontinence.

ABNORMALITY	DESCRIPTION
Senile dementia of Alzheimer disease	Subtle onset—generally with early memory loss—leading to severe deterioration in mental functions, profound disintegration of personality, and complete disorientation. Varied duration and rate of progression.
Seizure disorder	Episodic, sudden, violent, involuntary contractions of a group of muscles, with or without altering consciousness. Seizure can be partial or generalized and may be accompanied by urinary and fecal incontinence.
Meningitis	Fever, chills, nuchal rigidity, headache, seizures, and vomiting, followed by alterations in level of consciousness. **Can be life threatening.**
Encephalitis	Mild, febrile viral illness, often followed by a quiescent stage, then such CNS disturbances as headache, drowsiness, and confusion, leading to stupor and coma. Possible motor function impairment with severe paralysis or ataxia.
Lesions (intracranial)	Headaches, vomiting, change in cognition, motor dysfunction, seizures, and personality changes.
Cerebrovascular accident (stroke)	Sudden, focal neurologic deficit.

ABNORMALITY	DESCRIPTION
Parkinson disease	Initial symptoms: tremors at rest and with fatigue that disappear with movement and sleep. Progression: tremor of head; slowing of voluntary movement; bilateral pill-rolling of fingers; delays in execution of movement; masked facial expression; poor blink rate; short, shuffling steps; slowed, slurred, and monotonous speech; and possible behavioral changes and dementia.

CLINICAL SIGNS OF MOTOR NEURON LESIONS

Upper motor neuron	Lower motor neuron
Muscle spasticity, possible contractures	Muscle flaccidity
Little or no muscle atrophy, but decreased strength	Loss of muscle tone and strength; muscle atrophy
Hyperactive deep tendon and abdominal reflexes; absent plantar reflex	Weak or absent deep tendon, plantar, and abdominal reflexes
No fasciculations	Fasciculations
Damage above level of brainstem will affect opposite side of body	Changes in muscles supplied by that nerve, usually a muscle on same side as the lesion
Paralysis of lower part of face, if involved	Bell palsy, if face involved; coordination unimpaired

ABNORMALITY	DESCRIPTION
Mental retardation	Subaverage intellectual functioning, delayed development, inability to discriminate among stimuli, impaired short-term memory.
Cerebral palsy	Unexpected muscle tone, posture, motor performance, and reflexes.

SAMPLE DOCUMENTATION

Mental status. Appropriate dress and behavior. Oriented to time, place, and person. Reasoning and arithmetic calculations abilities intact. Immediate, recent, and remote memory intact. Appropriate mood and feeling expressed. Speech clearly and smoothly enunciated; comprehends direction.

Cranial nerves I-XII. Intact.

Proprioception and cerebellar function. Gait is coordinated and even. Romberg sign negative. Rapid alternating movements coordinated and smooth.

Sensory function. Superficial touch and pain sensation intact bilaterally.

Reflexes. Deep tendon reflex 2+ bilaterally in all extremities. Plantar reflex negative bilaterally; no clonus.

16

Head-to-Toe Examination

EXAMINATION OF THE ADULT

Because there is no one correct way to order the parts of the physical examination, you are encouraged to adapt the following suggested approach for a particular setting, patient condition, or patient disability.

General Inspection

Start the examination when the patient is within your view. As you first observe the patient, take note of the following:

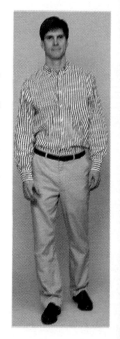

Signs of distress or disease
Habitus
Manner of sitting
Degree of relaxation on the face
Relationship with others in the room
Degree of interest in what is happening in the room
On greeting the patient, assess the following:
Alacrity with which you are met
Moistness of the palm when you shake hands
Eyes: luster and expression of emotion
Skin color
Facial expression
Mobility
    Use of assistive devices
    Gait
    Sitting, rising from chair
    Taking off coat
Dress and posture

Speech pattern, disorders, foreign language
Difficulty hearing, assistive devices
Stature and build
Musculoskeletal deformities
Vision problems, assistive devices
Eye contact with you
Orientation, mental alertness
Nutritional state
Respiratory problems
Significant others accompanying patient

Patient Instructions

Empty the bladder.
Remove as much clothing as is necessary.
Put on a gown.

Measurements

Measure height.
Measure weight.
Assess distance vision: Snellen chart.
Document vital signs: temperature, pulse, respiration, blood
    pressure in both arms.

Patient Seated, Wearing Gown

Stand in front of patient seated
    on examining table.

Head and face

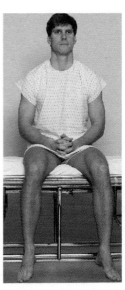

Inspect skin characteristics.
Inspect symmetry and external
    characteristics of eyes and
    ears.
Inspect configuration of skull.
Inspect and palpate scalp and
    hair for texture, distribution,
    and quantity of hair.
Palpate facial bones.
Palpate temporomandibular joint
    while patient opens and
    closes mouth.

Palpate sinus regions; if tender, transilluminate.

Inspect ability to clench teeth, squeeze eyes tightly shut, wrinkle forehead, smile, stick out tongue, puff out cheeks (CN V, VII).

Test light sensation of forehead, cheeks, chin (CN V).

Eyes

External examination:

Inspect eyelids, eyelashes, palpebral folds.

Determine alignment of eyebrows.

Inspect sclerae, conjunctivae, irides.

Palpate lacrimal apparatus.

Near vision screening: Rosenbaum chart (CN II).

Eye function:

Test pupillary response to light and accommodation.

Perform cover-uncover test and light reflex.

Test extraocular eye movements (CN III, IV, VI).

Assess visual fields (CN II).

Test corneal reflexes (CN V).

Ophthalmoscopic examination:

Test red reflex.

Inspect lens.

Inspect disc, cup margins, vessels, retinal surface, vitreous humor.

Ears

Inspect alignment.

Inspect surface characteristics.

Palpate auricle.

Assess hearing with whisper test or ticking watch (CN VIII).

Perform otoscopic examination:

Inspect canals.

Inspect tympanic membranes for landmarks, deformities, inflammation.

Use a tuning fork to assess bone and air conduction.

Nose

Note structure, position of septum.

Determine patency of each nostril.

Inspect mucosa, septum, and turbinates with nasal speculum.

Assess olfactory function when indicated: test sense of smell (CN I).

Mouth and pharynx

Inspect lips, buccal mucosa, gums, hard and soft palates, floor of mouth for color and surface characteristics.

Inspect oropharynx: note anteroposterior pillars, uvula, tonsils, posterior pharynx, mouth odor.

Inspect teeth for color, number, surface characteristics.

Inspect tongue for color, characteristics, symmetry, movement (CN XII).

Test gag reflex and "ah" reflex (CN IX, X).

Perform sense of taste test (CN VII and IX) when indicated.

Neck

Inspect for symmetry and smoothness of neck and thyroid.

Inspect for jugular venous distention.

Perform active and passive range of motion; test resistance against examiner's hand.

Test strength of shoulder shrug (CN IX).

Palpate carotid pulses. Be sure to palpate one side at a time.

Palpate tracheal position.

Palpate thyroid.

Palpate lymph nodes: preauricular and postauricular, occipital, tonsillar, submaxillary, submental, superficial cervical chain, posterior cervical, deep cervical, supraclavicular.

Auscultate carotid arteries and thyroid.

Upper extremities

Observe and palpate hands, arms, and shoulders.

Skin and nail characteristics

Muscle mass

Muscular strength

Musculoskeletal deformities

Joint range of motion: fingers, wrists, elbows, shoulders

Assess pulses: radial, brachial.

Palpate epitrochlear nodes.

Patient Seated, Back Exposed

Stand behind patient seated on examining table.

Have males pull gown down to the waist so the entire chest and back are exposed.

Have females expose back; keep breasts covered.

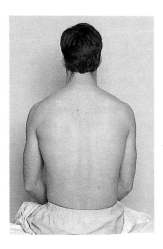

Back and posterior chest

Inspect skin and thoracic configuration.

Inspect symmetry of shoulders, musculoskeletal development.

Inspect and palpate scapulae and spine.

Palpate and percuss costovertebral angle.

Lungs

Inspect respiration: excursion, depth, rhythm, pattern.

Palpate for expansion and tactile fremitus.

Palpate scapular and subscapular nodes.

Percuss posterior chest and lateral walls systematically for resonance.

Percuss for diaphragmatic excursion.

Auscultate systematically for breath sounds (egophony, bronchophony, and whispered pectoriloquy): note characteristics and adventitious sounds.

Patient Seated, Chest Exposed

Move around to the front of the patient.
Have females lower gown to expose the anterior chest.

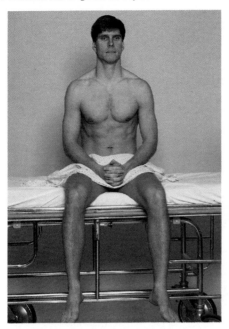

Anterior chest, lungs, and heart

Inspect skin, musculoskeletal development, symmetry.
Inspect respirations: patient posture, respiratory effort.
Inspect for pulsations or heaving.
Palpate chest wall for stability, crepitation, tenderness.
Palpate precordium for thrills, heaves, pulsations.
Palpate left chest to locate apical impulse.
Palpate for tactile fremitus.
Palpate nodes: infraclavicular, axillary.
Percuss systematically for resonance.
Auscultate systematically for breath sounds.
Auscultate systematically for heart sounds: aortic area, pulmonic area, second pulmonic area, tricuspid area, mitral area.

Female breasts

Inspect in these positions: patient's arms extended over head, pushing hands on hips, hands pushed together in front of chest, patient leaning forward.

Palpate breasts in all four quadrants, tail of Spence, over areolae; if breasts are large, perform bimanual palpation.

Palpate nipple: compress to observe for discharge.

Male breasts

Inspect breasts and nipples for symmetry, enlargement, surface characteristics.

Palpate breast tissue.

Patient Reclining 45 Degrees

Assist the patient to a reclining position at a 45-degree angle.

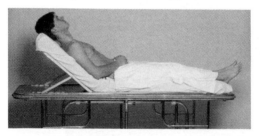

Stand to the side of the patient that allows the greatest comfort.

Inspect chest in recumbent position.

Inspect jugular venous pulsations and measure jugular venous pressure.

Patient Supine, Chest Exposed

Assist the patient into a supine position.

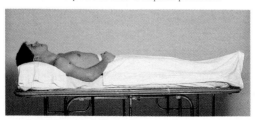

If the patient cannot tolerate lying flat, maintain head elevation at a 30-degree angle.

Uncover the chest while keeping the abdomen and lower extremities draped.

Female breasts

Inspect in recumbent position.

Palpate systematically with the patient's arm over her head and with her arm at her side.

Heart

Palpate the chest wall for thrills, heaves, pulsations.

Auscultate systematically; turn the patient slightly to the left side and repeat auscultation.

Patient Supine, Abdomen Exposed

Have the patient remain supine.

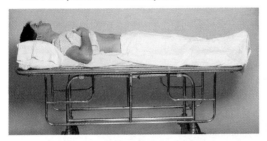

Cover the chest with the patient's gown.

Arrange draping to expose the abdomen from pubis to epigastrium.

Abdomen

Inspect skin characteristics, contour, pulsations, movement.

Auscultate all quadrants for bowel sounds.

Auscultate the aorta, renal arteries, and femoral arteries for bruits or venous hums.

Percuss all quadrants for tone.

Percuss liver borders and estimate span.

Percuss left midaxillary line for splenic dullness.

Lightly palpate all quadrants.

Deeply palpate all quadrants.

Palpate right costal margin for liver border.
Palpate left costal margin for spleen.
Palpate for right and left kidneys.
Palpate midline for aortic pulsation.
Test abdominal reflexes.
Have patient raise the head as you inspect the abdominal muscles.

Inguinal area

Palpate for lymph nodes, pulses, hernias.

External genitalia, males

Inspect penis, urethral meatus, scrotum, pubic hair.
Palpate scrotal contents (you may want to have the patient assume an alternate position, such as standing or sitting).

Patient Supine, Legs Exposed

Have patient remain supine.
Arrange drapes to cover the abdomen and pubis and to expose the lower extremities.

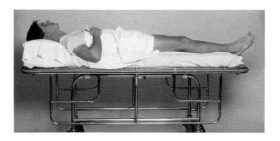

Feet and legs

Inspect for skin characteristics, hair distribution, muscle mass, musculoskeletal configuration.
Palpate for temperature, texture, edema, pulses (dorsalis pedis, posterior tibial, popliteal).
Test range of motion and strength of toes, feet, ankles, knees.

Hips

Palpate hips for stability.
Test range of motion and strength of hips.

Patient Sitting, Lap Draped

Assist the patient to a sitting position.
Have patient wear gown with a drape across the lap.

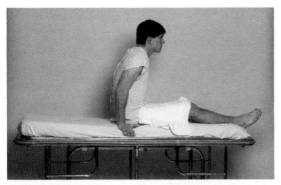

Musculoskeletal

Observe patient moving from lying to sitting position.
Note coordination, use of muscles, muscle strength, ease of
    movement.

Neurologic

Test sensory function: dull and sharp sensation of forehead,
    cheeks, chin, lower arms, hands, lower legs, feet.
Test vibratory sensation of wrists, ankles.
Test two-point discrimination of palms, thighs, back.
Test stereognosis, graphesthesia.
Test fine motor function, coordination, and position sense of
    upper extremities, asking patient to:
    Touch nose with alternating index fingers.
    Rapidly alternate touching fingers to thumb.
    Rapidly move index finger between own nose and examin-
        er's finger.
Test fine motor function, coordination, and position sense of
    lower extremities, asking patient to:
    Run heel down tibia of opposite leg.
    Alternately and rapidly cross leg over opposite knee.
Test deep tendon reflexes and compare bilaterally: biceps,
    triceps, brachioradial, patellar, Achilles.
Test the plantar reflex bilaterally.

Patient Standing

Assist patient to a standing position.
Stand next to patient.

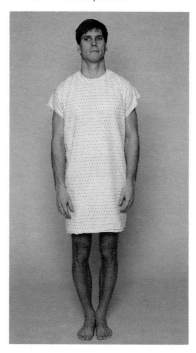

Spine

Inspect and palpate spine as patient bends over at waist.
Test range of motion: hyperextension, lateral bending, rotation of upper trunk.

Neurologic

Observe gait.
Test proprioception and cerebellar function:
    Perform Romberg test.
    Ask the patient to walk heel to toe.
    Ask the patient to stand on one foot, then the other, with eyes closed.

Ask the patient to hop in place on one foot, then the other.
Ask the patient to do deep knee bends.

Abdominal/genital

Test for inguinal and femoral hernias.

Female Patient, Lithotomy Position

Assist female patient into lithotomy position, and drape appropriately.
Sit next to patient.

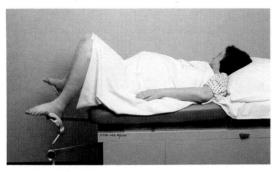

External genitalia

Inspect pubic hair, labia, clitoris, urethral opening, vaginal opening, perineal and perianal area, anus.
Palpate labia and Bartholin glands; milk Skene glands.

Internal genitalia

Perform speculum examination:
  Inspect vagina and cervix.
  Collect Pap smear and other necessary specimens.
Perform bimanual palpation to assess for characteristics of vagina, cervix, uterus, adnexae.
Perform rectovaginal examination to assess rectovaginal septum, broad ligaments.
Perform rectal examination:
  Assess anal sphincter tone and surface characteristics.
  Obtain rectal culture if needed.
  Note characteristics of stool when gloved finger is removed.

Male Patient, Bending Forward

Assist male patient in leaning over examining table or into knee-chest position. Stand behind patient.

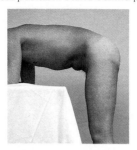

Inspect sacrococcygeal and perianal areas.

Perform rectal examination:

Palpate sphincter tone and surface characteristics.

Obtain rectal culture if needed.

Palpate prostate gland and seminal vesicles.

Note characteristics of stool when gloved finger is removed.

Conclude Examination

Allow patient to dress in private.

Share findings and interpretations with patient.

Answer any of the patient's additional questions.

Confirm that the patient has a clear understanding of all aspects of the situation.

If the patient is examined in a hospital bed:

Put everything back in order when finished.

Make sure the patient is comfortably settled in an appropriate manner.

Put bed side rails up if the clinical condition warrants it.

Make sure that buttons and buzzers are within easy reach.

EXAMINATION OF THE CHILD

Take child's temperature, weight, and length or height.

Offer toys or paper and pencil to entertain the child, to develop rapport, and to evaluate development, motor and neurologic status.

Use a developmental screening test such as the Denver II to evaluate language, motor coordination, and social skills.

Evaluate mental status as the child interacts with you and with the parent.

Take advantage of opportunities the child presents during the examination to make your observations.

Child Playing

While the child plays on the floor, evaluate the musculoskeletal and neurologic systems while developing a rapport with the child.

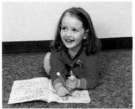

Observe the child's spontaneous activities.

Ask the child to demonstrate skills such as throwing a ball, building block towers, drawing geometric figures, coloring.

Evaluate gait, jumping, hopping, range of motion.

Muscle strength: Observe the child climbing on the parent's lap, stooping and recovering.

Child on Parent's Lap

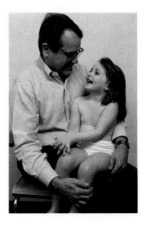

Perform the examination on the parent's lap to enhance the child's participation.

Begin with the child sitting and undressed except for the diaper or underpants.

Upper extremities

Inspect arms for movement, size, shape; observe use of the hands; inspect hands for number and configuration of fingers, palmar creases.

Palpate radial pulses.

Elicit biceps and triceps reflexes when child cooperates.

Take blood pressure at this point or later, depending on child's attitude.

Lower extremities

Child may stand for much or part of the examination.

Inspect legs for movement, size, shape, alignment, lesions.

Inspect feet for alignment, longitudinal arch, number of toes.

Palpate dorsalis pedis pulse.

Elicit plantar reflex and, if child is cooperative, the Achilles and patellar reflexes.

Head and neck

Inspect head:

Inspect shape, alignment with neck, hairline, position of auricles.

Palpate anterior fontanel for size; head for sutures, depressions; hair for texture.

Measure head circumference.

Inspect neck for webbing, voluntary movement.

Palpate neck: position of trachea, thyroid, muscle tone, lymph nodes.

Chest, heart, and lungs

Inspect the chest for respiratory movement, size, shape, precordial movement, deformity, nipple and breast development.

Palpate the anterior chest, locate the point of maximal impulse, note tactile fremitus in the talking or crying child.

Auscultate the anterior, lateral, and posterior chest for breath sounds; count respirations.

Auscultate all cardiac listening areas for S_1 and S_2, splitting, and murmurs; count apical pulse.

Child Relatively Supine, Still on Lap, Diaper Loosened

Inspect abdomen:

Auscultate for bowel sounds.

Palpate: identify size of the liver and any other palpable organs or masses.

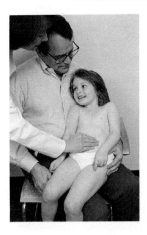

Percuss.

Palpate the femoral pulses, compare to radial pulses.

Palpate for lymph nodes.

Inspect the external genitalia.

Males: palpate scrotum for descent of testes and other masses.

Child Standing

Inspect spinal alignment as the child bends slowly forward to touch toes.

Observe posture from anterior, posterior, and lateral views.

Observe gait.

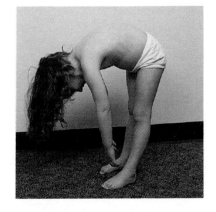

Child on Parent's Lap
Prepare child for examination

Only if absolutely necessary, restrain the child for funduscopic, otoscopic, and oral examinations.

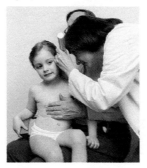

Lessen the fear of these examinations by permitting the child to handle the instruments, blow out the light, or use them on a doll or on the parent.

Attempt to gain the child's cooperation, even if it takes more time; future visits will be more pleasant for both of you.

After finishing these preliminary maneuvers, perform the following:

  Inspect eyes: corneal light reflex, red reflex, extraocular movements, funduscopic examination.

  Perform otoscopic examination.

  Inspect nasal mucosa.

  Inspect mouth and pharynx.

(NOTE: By the time the child is of school age, it is usually possible to use an examination sequence very similar to that for adults.) See pp. 234-241 for examples of forms used to chart physical growth.

EXAMINATION OF THE PREGNANT WOMAN

Use the same process of physical examination as for the adult.

In addition, perform more extensive abdominal and pelvic evaluations for pregnancy status and fetal well-being.

Late in pregnancy, a woman may find it difficult to assume the supine position without experiencing hypotension; use this position only when necessary.

Provide alternative positioning by elevating the backrest, or by supplying pillows for the woman to assume the left side-lying position.

Have her empty her bladder to make the abdominal assessment more comfortable for her and more accurate.

Remember that during pregnancy, urinary urgency and frequency are common.

GIRLS: BIRTH TO 36 MONTHS
PHYSICAL GROWTH
NCHS PERCENTILES*

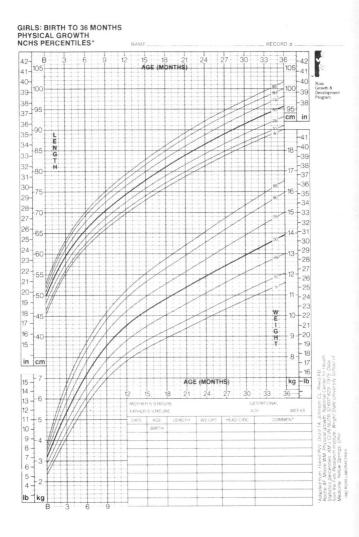

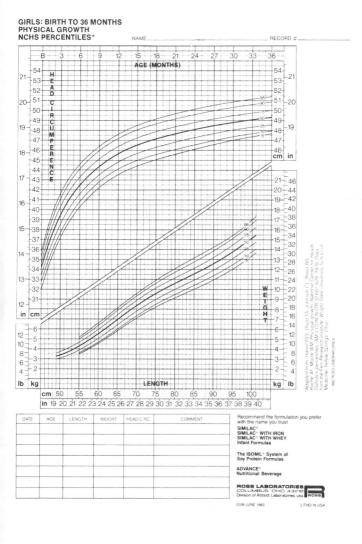

GIRLS: BIRTH TO 36 MONTHS
PHYSICAL GROWTH
NCHS PERCENTILES*

NAME _____   RECORD # _____

BOYS: BIRTH TO 36 MONTHS
PHYSICAL GROWTH
NCHS PERCENTILES*

NAME _____   RECORD # _____

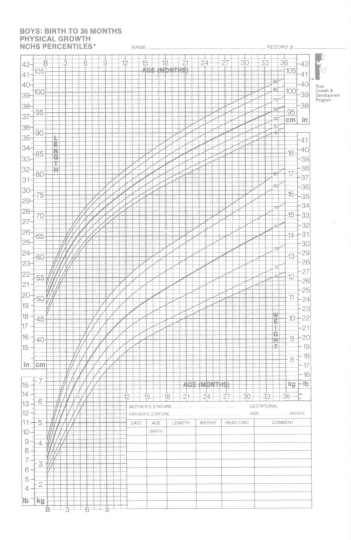

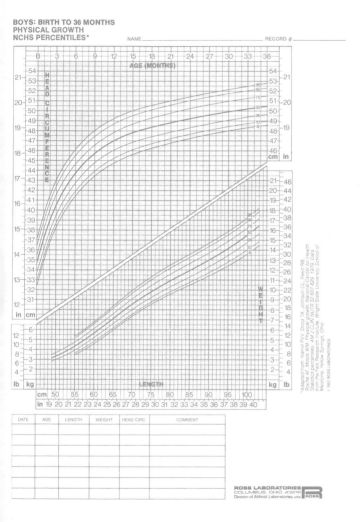

GIRLS: 2 TO 18 YEARS
PHYSICAL GROWTH
NCHS PERCENTILES*

NAME _____   RECORD # _____

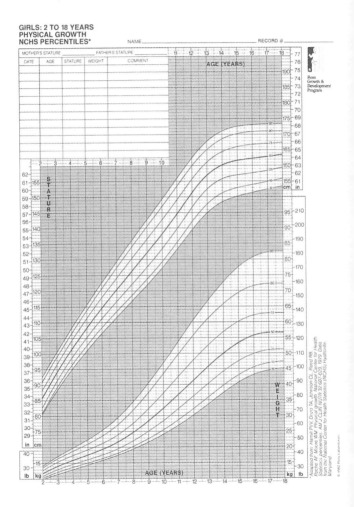

Ross Growth & Development Program

*Adapted from: Hamill PVV, Drizd TA, Johnson CL, Reed RB, Roche AF, Moore WM. Physical growth: National Center for Health Statistics percentiles. AM J CLIN NUTR 32:607-629, 1979. Data from the National Center for Health Statistics (NCHS), Hyattsville, Maryland.

GIRLS: PREPUBESCENT
PHYSICAL GROWTH
NCHS PERCENTILES*

NAME _____

RECORD # _____

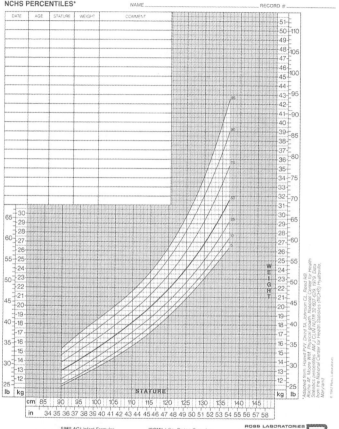

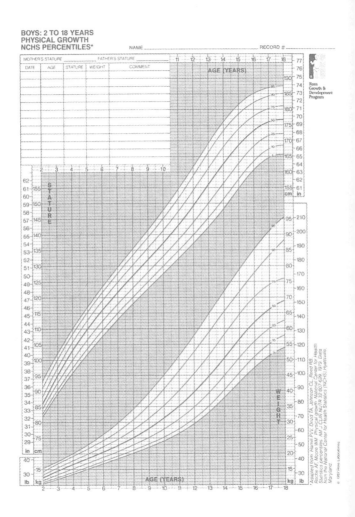

BOYS: 2 TO 18 YEARS
PHYSICAL GROWTH
NCHS PERCENTILES*

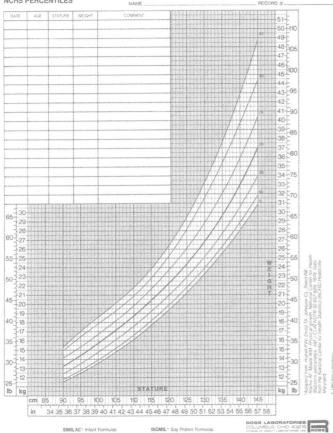

BOYS: PREPUBESCENT
PHYSICAL GROWTH
NCHS PERCENTILES*

17

Reporting and Recording

THE HISTORY

Record the patient's history, especially in an initial visit, to provide a comprehensive data base. Arrange information appropriately in specific categories, usually in a particular sequence. Use the following organized sequence as a guide.

Identifying Information

Patient's name
Identification number
Age
Marital status
Address
Phone numbers
Occupation
Date of visit
For children and dependent adults, names of parents or next of kin
Put identifying information on each page of record.

Source and Reliability of Information

Document who is giving the history and the relationship to patient.
Indicate when an old record is used.
State judgment about the reliability of the information.

Chief Complaint

Reason the patient sought health care, in patient's own words or paraphrased (only if this makes the complaint more clear).
State symptoms only, not a premature diagnosis.

Present Problem

List and describe current symptoms of the chief complaint and their appearance chronologically in reverse order.

List any expected symptoms that are absent.

Note pertinent information from the review of systems, family history, and personal/social history along with findings.

Where more than one problem is identified, address each in a separate paragraph, including the following details of symptom occurrence:

Time intervals: time of day, duration, and changes in symptoms over time.

Character or quality: severity, location and nature, as for pain.

Association with certain events: eating, activity, rest.

Treatments: those attempted and the outcome.

Interference with activities of daily living.

Current medications: both prescription and nonprescription, dosage and schedule.

Past Medical History

List and describe each of the following, with dates of occurrence and any specific information available:

Hospitalizations and illnesses: surgery, injuries, and disabilities, major childhood and adult illnesses.

Previous health care: include past health examinations, immunizations, laboratory studies, obstetric care.

Allergies: especially to drugs, previous transfusion reactions, and to other substances.

Family History

Present information about the age and health of family members in narrative or genogram form.

Family members: include parents, grandparents, aunts and uncles, siblings, spouse, and children. For deceased family members, note the age at time of death and cause, if known.

Major health or genetic disorders: include hypertension, cancer, cardiac, respiratory, renal, cerebrovascular or thyroid disorders, asthma or other allergic manifestations, blood dyscrasias, psychiatric difficulties, tuberculosis, diabetes mellitus, hepatitis or other familial disorders.

Personal/Social History

Include information according to the concerns of the patient and the influence of the health problem on the patient's life:

Cultural background.

Family structure: who is at home, stresses, personal problems, events of a typical day, sources of strength, the impact of the health problem or the family's response to illness.

Educational and economic status.

Environment: home, school, work, structural barriers if handicapped, community services utilized.

Current health habits or risk factors: exercise, smoking, alcohol intake, salt intake, weight control.

Review of Systems

Organize in a general head-to-toe sequence, including an impression of each symptom.

Record expected or negative findings as the absence of symptoms or problems.

When unexpected or positive findings are stated by the patient, include details from further inquiry as you would in the present illness.

Include the following categories of information (sequence may vary):

General constitutional symptoms
Nutrition
Skin, hair, and nails
Lymphatic
Head and neck
Eyes, ears, nose, and throat (EENT)
Breasts
Heart and blood vessels
Chest and lungs
Endocrine
Immunologic
Hematologic
Gastrointestinal
Genitourinary
Musculoskeletal
Neurologic
Psychiatric

PHYSICAL FINDINGS
General Statement

Age, race, sex, general appearance

Nutritional status, weight, height, and body mass index

Vital signs: temperature, pulse rate, respiratory rate, blood pressure

Communication skills, behavior, awareness, orientation, co-operation with examination

Skin

Color, integrity, temperature, hydration

Presence of edema, excessive perspiration, unusual odor

Presence and description of lesions (inflammation, tenderness, induration, discharge, parasites, trauma)

Hair texture and distribution

Nail configuration, color, texture, condition, presence of clubbing

Head

Size and contour of head, scalp appearance

Symmetry and spacing of facial features

Presence of edema or puffiness

Temporal arteries: characteristics

Eyes

Visual acuity, visual fields

Appearance of orbits, conjunctivae, sclerae, eyelids, eyebrows

Extraocular movements, pupillary shape, consensual response to light and accommodation, corneal light reflex, cover-uncover test

Ophthalmoscopic findings of cornea, lens, retina, optic disc, macula, retinal vessel size, caliber and arteriovenous (AV) crossings

Ears

Configuration, position and alignment of auricles

Otoscopic findings of canals (cerumen, discharge, foreign body) and tympanic membranes (integrity, color, landmarks, mobility)

Hearing: Air and bone conduction tests

Nose

Appearance of external nose, nasal patency
Presence of discharge, crusting, flaring, polyp
Appearance of turbinates, alignment of septum
Presence of sinus tenderness or swelling
Discrimination of odors

Mouth and Throat

Number, occlusion and condition of teeth; presence of dental appliances
Appearance of lips, tongue, buccal and oral mucosa, and floor of mouth (color, moisture, surface characteristics, symmetry)
Appearance of pharynx, tonsils, palate
Symmetry and movement of tongue, soft palate and uvula; gag reflex
Discrimination of taste
Voice quality

Neck

Mobility, suppleness, and strength
Position of trachea
Thyroid size, shape, and tenderness
Presence of masses

Chest

Size and shape of chest, anteroposterior diameter, symmetry of movement with respiration
Presence of retractions, use of accessory muscles
Diaphragmatic movement

Lungs

Respiratory rate, depth, regularity, quietness or ease of respiration
Palpation findings: symmetry and quality of tactile fremitus
Percussion findings: quality and symmetry of percussion notes, difference in diaphragm level on inspiration and expiration
Auscultation findings: characteristics of breath sounds (vesicular, bronchial, bronchiovesicular, adventitious), phase and location where audible

Characteristics of cough
Presence of friction rub, egophony, whispered pectoriloquy or bronchophony

Breasts

Size, shape
Symmetry, presence of masses, scars, tenderness, thickening, discharge or dimpling
Characteristics of nipples and areolae

Heart

Anatomic location of apical impulse
Heart rate, rhythm, amplitude, contour, and symmetry of apical impulse and pulse in extremities
Blood pressure: comparison between extremities, with position change
Palpation findings: pulsations, thrills, heaves, or lifts
Auscultation findings: characteristics of S_1 and S_2 (location, intensity, pitch, timing, splitting, systole, diastole)
Presence of murmurs, clicks, snaps, S_3 or S_4 (timing, location, radiation intensity, pitch, quality)

Blood Vessels

Jugular vein distention and pressure measurement
Presence of bruits over carotid, temporal, renal, and femoral arteries, abdominal aorta
Temperature, color, hair distribution, skin texture, nail beds of lower extremities
Presence of edema, swelling, vein distention, Homan sign, or tenderness of lower extremities

Abdomen

Shape, contour, visible aorta pulsations
Auscultation findings: bowel sounds in all quadrants, their character
Palpation findings: aorta, organs, feces, masses, location, size, contour, consistency, tenderness
Percussion findings: areas of different percussion notes, costovertebral angle (CVA) tenderness
Liver span

Male Genitalia

Appearance of external genitalia, circumcision status, location and size of urethral opening, discharge, lesions, distribution of pubic hair

Palpation findings: penis, testes, epididymides, vasa deferentia, contour, consistency, tenderness

Presence of hernia or scrotal swelling

Female Genitalia

Appearance of external genitalia and perineum, distribution of pubic hair, tenderness, scarring, discharge

Internal examination findings: appearance of vaginal mucosa, cervix, discharge, odor

Bimanual examination findings: size, tenderness of cervix, uterus, adnexae, and ovaries

Rectovaginal examination findings

Anus, Rectum

Sphincter control, presence of hemorrhoids, fissures, skin tags

Rectal wall contour, tenderness

Prostate size, contour, consistency

Color and consistency of stool

Lymphatic

Presence of lymph nodes in neck, epitrochlear, axillary or inguinal areas

Size, shape, tenderness, mobility, discreetness of nodes

Musculoskeletal

Posture: alignment of extremities and spine, symmetry of body parts

Symmetry of muscle mass, tone and strength; grading of strength

Range of motion, passive and active; presence of pain with movement

Appearance of joints; presence of deformities, tenderness or crepitus

Neurologic

Mental status: orientation; reasoning and calculations; memory, mood, and feelings; speech clarity; comprehension; mental status examination score

Cranial nerves: specific findings for each or specify those tested, if findings are recorded in head and neck sections

Cerebellar and motor function: gait, balance, coordination with rapid alternating motions

Sensory function, symmetry

Superficial and deep tendon reflexes: symmetry, grade

REFERENCES

Bobak I, Jensen N, Zalar M: *Maternity and gynecologic care: the nurse and the family*, ed 5, St Louis, 1993, Mosby.

Folstein MF, Folstein SE, McHugh PR: "Mini-Mental State": a practical method for grading the cognitive state of patients for the clinician, J *Psychiatr Res* 12:189, 1975.

Habif T: *Clinical dermatology: a color guide to diagnosis and therapy*, ed 2, St Louis, 1990, Mosby.

Judge R, Zuidema G, Fitzgerald F: *Clinical diagnosis*, ed 5, Boston, 1988, Little, Brown.

Malasanos L, Barkauskas V, Stoltenberg-Allen K: *Health assessment*, ed 4, St Louis, 1990, Mosby.

McCarty DJ: *Arthritis and allied conditions: a textbook of rheumatology*, ed 2, Philadelphia, 1993, Lea & Febiger.

Proffit WR et al: *Contemporary orthodontics*, ed 2, St Louis, 1993, Mosby.

Rudy EB: *Advanced neurological and neurosurgical nursing*, St Louis, 1984, Mosby.

Thompson JM et al: *Mosby's clinical nursing*, ed 3, St Louis, 1993, Mosby.

Wong DL: *Whaley & Wong's nursing care of infants and children*, ed 5, St Louis, 1995, Mosby.

Index

V

U

W